W9-BSN-547

THE AMERICAN YOGA ASSOCIATION'S BEGINNER'S MANUAL

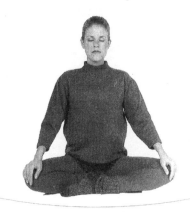

Alice Christensen

A FIRESIDE BOOK

Published by Simon & Schuster

New York London Toronto Sydney Singapore

FIRESIDE
Rockefeller Center
1230 Avenue of the Americas
New York, NY 10020

For information about special discounts for bulk purchases,
please contact Simon & Schuster Special Sales: 1-800-456-6798 or business@simonandschuster.com

Designed by Jill Weber

Manufactured in the United States of America

1   3   5   7   9   10   8   6   4   2

Library of Congress Cataloging-in-Publication Data
Christensen, Alice.
The American Yoga Association's beginner's manual / Alice Christensen
p.   cm.
"A Fireside book."
1. Yoga, Hatha.   I. Title.
RA781.7.C48635 2002
613.7'046–dc21   2001040748
ISBN 0-7432-1941-4

Some of the material in this book is based on *The Light of Yoga Society's Beginner's Manual.*

The techniques, ideas, and suggestions presented in this book are not intended to substitute for proper medical advice. Consult your physician before beginning this or any new exercise program. The author, the American Yoga Association, and the publisher assume no responsibility for injuries suffered while practicing these techniques. If you are pregnant or nursing, consult your physician about which techniques you can safely perform. If you are elderly or have any chronic or recurring conditions, such as high blood pressure, neck or back pain, arthritis, or heart disease, seek your physician's advice about which program to follow. The American Yoga Association does not recommend Yoga asans for children under age sixteen.

Photographs of asans and techniques by Evelyn England, SAGE Productions, Sarasota, Florida. The models for this book are Krista Benz, Patrick Benz, Steve Ellis, Anne Ferrier, Artie Guerin, Carole Guerin, G. Q. Haze, Lea Jackson, Steven Sanchez, and Margaret Toward.

ALSO BY
Alice Christensen

Acknowledgments

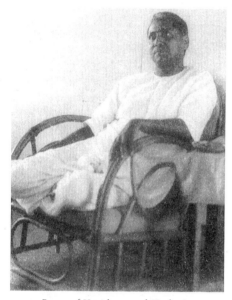

*Rama of Haridwar and Kashmir,
India (1900–1972)*

The following people have been a great help in producing the revised edition of this book: Pattie Cerar, who provided constant support with innumerable details; Linda Gajevski, whose creative direction was invaluable during the entire project; Stephen Grant, who researched the complexities of current nutritional thought and formed them into a coherent chapter; and Patricia Rockwood, who supplied able editorial assistance throughout the writing process. I would also like to thank our editor at Simon & Schuster, Lisa Considine, who directed our revision with tact and insight, and the art director, Cherlynne Li, and designer, Mary Ann Smith, who produced a beautiful book with clean, contemporary styling.

This book is dedicated to Rama, the source of my expression of Yoga in the world.

CONTENTS

PREFACE

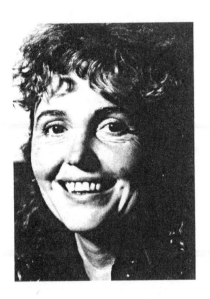

It has been nearly thirty years since we published the very first edition of this book, in 1972, and nearly fifteen since the second, in 1987. Although all of us have grown and changed over the years, it is a testament to the enduring power of Yoga that its expression in the world is stronger than ever. Yoga is interpreted and taught in so many different ways, from the athleticism of some groups to the meditative emphasis of others. Yoga itself stays the same, offering timeless techniques for self-discovery that all can welcome into their lives. I hope that you find this new edition useful in your personal search for meaning in life.

Yoga was not a popular subject in the United States when it first entered my life in the early fifties. I did not consciously seek Yoga, as many people do today. Rather, Yoga came to me with the suddenness of a vision one summer night and turned my life upside down.

I awoke out of a sound sleep to see a huge column of white light at the foot of my bed. Its radiance filled the room, reminding me of the intense light of downed power lines. I drew myself back against the headboard, terrified, but I could not speak or cry out. I knew that I was not dreaming, because I was aware of the curtains billowing softly at the open window and the maple tree waving gently outside in the summer breeze. I watched and waited, suddenly very quiet, as the light advanced toward me, covered me, and seemed to enter me. I lost consciousness and awoke in the morning at my usual time. But as I got out of bed and started to dress, the word *Yoga* sprang into my mind. I had heard the word only once before, at the annual county fair, where one of the curiosities was a turbaned man who claimed to be able to foretell the future.

My life did not change much at first, except for the push of that word *Yoga* in the back of my mind. I tried to approach the subject with other people, in roundabout ways, but I found no one who knew any more than I did. I found that it would not go away, so I started to read everything I could get my hands on in order to learn more about Yoga. I wrote to every Yoga teacher and organization whose address I could find—but none of my letters was answered. My life became more and more unsettling. I became clairvoyant. I started to dream in foreign languages and to have visions of strange people talking to me, teaching me.

One man came more and more often in the visions and dreams; he was Sivananda, then living at Rishikesh, in India. He began appearing to me at odd times, usually at the kitchen sink while I was doing dishes. At first I would run out of the room in fright. But eventually I lost my fear and my resistance to this upheaval in my life, and Sivananda began teaching me in earnest. Each day I spent several hours reading and studying, trying to meditate and learn the asans that I read about.

Yoga gave me tremendous concentration, and I found that I could continue to manage a large house and take care of my family even better than before. I became very efficient. Sorting out all the things in my life that I felt were not necessary, I settled down to concentrate on what had meaning for me and for those around me.

Sivananda taught me the beginnings of the techniques that have become the backbone of my life and thought. He provided constant and sympathetic help for several years during my search to find the meaning of Yoga in my life, and I am still grateful to him. Just as I was making plans to go to India to meet him, I heard that Sivananda had died. Devastated, I tried to give up my Yoga practices, only to find myself irresistibly drawn back to Yoga and to its promises of health, peace, stability, and true happiness in my life. I had found a wonderful acceptance in myself of who I was and what I could become, and the steadiness and support of that knowledge gave me the strength to continue what I knew I must do.

I kept on practicing, on my own, until I met Rama of Kashmir and Haridwar, India, the next year. He was brought to this country by a group of people in Cleveland, where I lived. An Indian student of Rama's was working at Case Western Reserve University in Cleveland. Somehow he found out that I was practicing Yoga, and he invited me to go with him to meet Rama at the airport. I watched a beautiful brown man in a Kashmiri bathrobe step off the airplane. He walked straight over to me and said, "Alice, I have come to get you." Rama accepted me as a student and became the teacher and guide that I had been looking for all the years before. His love, inspiration, and wisdom led me through the training I needed to progress in Yoga. Yoga had become a certainty in my life.

With Rama's guidance, the Light of Yoga Society (now known as the American Yoga Association) was formed in 1968 as a vehicle to make the benefits of Yoga more easily accessible to people in this part of the world. Rama oversaw the publication of the first edition of this book in 1972. Since that time I have seen many of his dreams taking shape as more and more people come to realize the freedom that Yoga practice can bring about.

I have always wanted freedom: the freedom to find and to be myself; to do what I want to do in life and what I feel I must do. Yoga has given me that freedom. I no longer feel imprisoned by my fears, by ill health, or by turbulent emotional swings. I no longer feel unable to communicate or to love. Yoga has enabled me to reach and explore new levels of awareness, so that my entire outlook on life has changed. I am happier now than I have ever been.

My life is never boring. In all the years that have passed since that brilliant light first entered my life, I have been showered with the richness of new insight and experience. The results of my practice and my teaching have not always been what I expected, but they have always been what I most needed. Yoga has helped me attain peace of mind, strength, inspiration, and energy, which we all need for living a full, useful, and happy life.

Before Rama died he directed me to continue my studies with the great master Lakshmanjoo in Srinagar, Kashmir, and, to my great good fortune, Lakshmanjoo accepted me as his student. This wonderful man, revered in India as a saint, was the only living master of a complex branch of Yoga called Kashmir Shaivism. Lakshmanjoo, who died in 1991, gave me the precious opportunity to continue being a student of Yoga; eventually, the ability to continue learning becomes a necessity.

My relationship with my teachers was very different from what I see around me in the many Yoga programs being offered in the Western world these days. I hardly ever asked my great teachers a direct question about Yoga, and what I needed to know was hardly ever conveyed to me in words. Once, when I told Rama about a strange experience that had happened to me, his response was simply "That means something." On the rare occasions

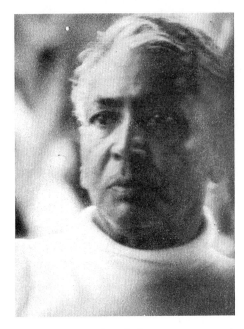

when I ventured to ask Lakshmanjoo a question, he would often answer with an apparently unrelated comment, such as "Isn't the garden beautiful today?" or "Doesn't that bird's song taste delicious?" turning me back into my own thought.

After years of teaching Yoga myself, I am beginning to understand the limitations of language. It's difficult to write a book about Yoga that conveys the type of teaching that has supported me all these years. I am delving deeper into the Tantric approach, where words become coarse and everything becomes feeling, which is the language of the inner emotional-spiritual body. *Yoga* means "union"—the joining of the outer physical body to the inner emotional-spiritual body. I hope that as you read the words in this book, you will think of them as a kind of shell, a structure holding the secret of inspiration that will help you to recognize the many possibilities in your thoughts and emotions that are beyond language. These will be offered to you as you recognize and encourage your inner body to express itself.

In 1972, when the first edition of this book was published, our aim was to offer a clear and practical guide for people who were interested in learning about Yoga. The seventies were a time for trying out the many new attitudes and lifestyles that seemed to offer a healthier and more fulfilling way of life than was customary. Yoga is one method of creating a sense of well-being that began as a fad but now has become recognized and appreciated as a dependable self-help source. Although very few people may feel drawn to practice Yoga as intensively as I do, many more are beginning to recognize how even a few Yoga techniques, practiced regularly, can help us address the challenges and problems we face today.

Our world has become increasingly complex, filled with dismaying problems such as famine, poverty, and injustice, whose magnitude can inspire real feelings of helplessness. While we may often feel overwhelmed in the face of such global concerns, we can make a difference, starting with ourselves. As we improve our health and become creative, productive, and aware of our motives, we can learn to take responsibility for the effects of our actions, thoughts, and desires. We become whole, happier with ourselves and with the challenges of daily life. Our personal examples cannot help but affect our families, friends, and co-workers. This will ensure a richer, happier life for our communities and our world.

This book will teach you how to use Yoga techniques to help make your life happier and more fulfilling. I wish you the best of success as you begin your adventure of Yoga. You'll need faith in the unknown and a willingness to wait as long as it takes—a quality that is foreign to our Western demand for instant gratification. I encourage you to try it; I am finding great joy in the journey. As my teachers used to say, "What else do you have to do?"

Alice Christensen
SARASOTA, FLORIDA

Chapter 1

INTRODUCTION TO YOGA

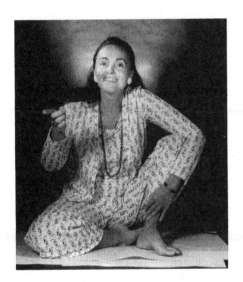

Yoga is a step-by-step process that brings health, self-awareness, and self-fulfillment. That process employs techniques that bring together the outer, physical body and the inner, emotional-spiritual body in complete, balanced strength.

The word *Yoga* comes from the Sanskrit root *yug,* which means "to join together" or "to yoke." Yoga ends the separateness that can exist internally, between different aspects of yourself, and externally, between yourself and the world. The practice of Yoga brings the disparate aspects of the body, mind, and personality into balance so that you end up with a strength and clarity of purpose that is supported by your whole being.

Yoga describes individual human existence as having two bodies: the inner emotional-spiritual body and the outer physical body. Normally, the physical dominates, meaning that most of our worldly efforts are fueled with but half our potential strength. By encouraging the inner body to balance with the outer body, the individual gains great peace and power. When we are able to yoke the outer and inner bodies together, we reach full potential. Try to imagine your efforts at full strength—amplifying your power by a factor of two. This has always been the goal of Yoga. Bringing the two halves of the personality together in balance and harmony produces a powerful, ethical, balanced person with extraordinary ability.

Most of us can never state clearly why we want to start to practice Yoga. Classic books on the subject all refer to a type of time clock, set within us at birth, that begins the process that leads, after many lifetimes, to the search for Yoga. People come to Yoga classes with various goals, ranging from learning a few simple stress management techniques to investigating the workings of their own minds. I often ask students who come to me, "Why have you come here? What do you want?" And they usually state goals relating to health, or good sleep, and sometimes, echoing the marketing of Yoga in our country, they come to be beautiful and retain their youthful appearance. But all eventually look to heal the separateness they feel within themselves.

The adaptability of Yoga's techniques makes it possible to achieve a variety of goals while creating new, spontaneous support for future development. The great force of Yoga is not perceived in the beginning, but with daily practice it begins to emerge from the inner body. Students who so innocently expected limited results become conscious of deep and subtle thought, and the inner body provides a new awareness of a part of themselves that they had not realized before.

You can achieve your goals if you are willing to practice regularly. Ten minutes a day will produce immediate results. Yoga techniques can be used to build concentrated, directed strength. No matter what your background, a program of regular practice will enhance your life. You will notice a marked difference in your physical and mental outlook in as little as two weeks. You'll notice new confidence and enhanced well-being, and soon the practice will become addictive. You won't want to feel any other way. Because of this, very few people ever stop their practice once they establish a routine. Many exercise programs become boring and painful after some length of time. This is not the case with Yoga practice. You will find that your body and mind long for it, and although you do much the same routine every day, it has a strong, comforting effect on both your physical self and your emotional being.

Fortunately, many of us devote concentrated attention to our inner emotional-spiritual body. People have become much more accepting of the search for meaning within themselves, and they are discovering that they cannot be happy without a connection to their inner emotional-spiritual natures. When the emotional and physical bodies become balanced, the result is real power and happiness. Yoga asans, pranayamas (breathing exercises), and meditation all invite the inner emotional-spiritual body to speak. When this happens, intuitive and creative processes flourish effortlessly, supplying enormous verve and joy in life and work.

THE TECHNIQUES OF YOGA

Yoga techniques focus the breath and the mind and encourage completeness in the individual through ethical practice, physical exercises (asans), breathing techniques (pranayama), and meditation training.

Yoga asans (exercises) are designed to develop maximum flexibility and strength in the skeletal, muscular, and nervous systems, with special emphasis on building a strong and supple spine. The movement of asans massages the internal organs and improves circulation, causing the release and distribution of vital hormones as well as supplying the brain and every cell in your body with more oxygen and health-building nutrients. Muscles relax and heal more easily. A gradual strengthening of the nervous system builds concentration, poise, and a stronger connection with the inner body. In fact, the classical books on Yoga state that the purpose of Yoga asans is not simply to reap physical benefits (as it is presented in many classes in the West today) but rather to bring the body to utmost health and strength so that the practitioner can focus on meditation without distraction.

Yoga breathing exercises are very effective in helping you cope with stress, increase your energy level, and recover from fatigue. Controlled breathing also helps to relax mental turbulence. Proper breathing practice enhances concentration and improves memory.

Meditation practice helps you to quiet mental conversation with yourself as well as the emotional issues that constantly crowd your mind. Regular practice will enhance your ability to relax at will. Yoga students also find that meditation helps to release dormant powers of intuition and creative methods of problem solving.

As I mentioned previously, the techniques of Yoga can help you achieve a variety of goals and enhance your lifestyle. For this reason, in addition to the basic Yoga curriculum, we have included discussions of the Yogic approach to nutrition, some special techniques for stress management, routines for athletes and pregnant women, and a chapter that introduces our ethics-based approach to Yoga philosophy. A successful Yoga program depends heavily upon strong attention to ethical behavior, which will support and enhance your personal practice.

Yoga is not a religion, though many world religions have incorporated Yoga techniques because their practice provides a ready access to our inner emotional-spiritual selves. Many people are confused by the relationship between Yoga and Hinduism, and often mistakenly believe Yoga to be a part of the Hindu philosophy. Not so! Yoga actually predates Hinduism. Joseph Campbell, in his wonderful four-volume series *The Masks of God,* makes the distinction clear. The fact is, no one knows where or when Yoga began. It has always been there, and it is unique in offering a tradition of physical and psychological processes that lead to self-discovery. Yoga's extensive ethical system provides a strong foundation of spiritual values that many find refreshing in our chaotic world.

BEFORE YOU START

Always check with your doctor before starting any new exercise program, especially if you have not exercised regularly in several years. If you have physical constraints such as high blood pressure, heart disease, arthritis, or spinal disk injuries, consult with your physician about the program you choose. Do not embark on a program if you have had surgery within the last two months, until you have checked with your doctor.

What to Expect

Most people notice minor soreness when they are beginning a new exercise program, especially if they've been inactive for a long time. However, pain in your back, legs, or joints may indicate that you are straining yourself. Follow the instructions carefully so that your experience of Yoga will be safe and enjoyable.

Even if you have practiced Yoga before, we suggest that you start with the introductory routine for several weeks before launching into more difficult routines. Beginners often experience an initial elation when they start to practice Yoga on a regular basis. Chemical changes, such as the release of endorphins in the brain, occur during any sustained exercise program. The special combination of movement, breathing, and concentration that is unique to Yoga will encourage a comfortable assimilation of these changes. Be careful not to let your enthusiasm lead to straining yourself beyond your capacity. Set reasonable goals, both for the rate at which you progress and for the amount of time you commit to practice each day. Protect your body from self-violence.

Warm up for at least 5 minutes before you go on to your first routine. Read through each exercise in Chapter 2 before you try it. If you have to work around a physical constraint, you may need to modify the exercise in order to perform it comfortably. Move slowly and deliberately, and do not strain. You'll enhance the benefits of asans by coordinating physical movements with a steady breath pattern, and by maintaining concentration.

I have noticed that some teachers try to set a speed and endurance approach to asans. This approach can cause serious problems, turning some students away from Yoga altogether. Yoga is not a competitive sport. On the contrary, it is most effective when practiced in silence and alone. Forcing movements to the point of strain or pain is self-destructive, which is totally against the precept of Nonviolence, a basic ethic of Yoga practice. Don't let your mind force your physical body into something it doesn't want to do. The inner emotional-spiritual body must be coaxed to show its hand, and violence is not productive.

Chapter 3 introduces suggested course progressions. Find your own pace. The weekly routines are only suggestions. If you are elderly, have physical limitations, or are in drug or alcohol recovery, give your body time to get used to the movements. You may have to simplify the positions to some degree. Be creative. Yoga is not a rigid process but a fluid one, allowing every individual to find his or her proper pace and intensity. Eventually you will be able to assume the full, proper poses.

Competition is a word destructive to successful Yoga practice. Try to think of your progress as isolated from what others are doing. Don't compare yourself critically with anyone else or the models who demonstrate the asans in this book. The important thing is that you set and keep a regular practice time.

Similarly, do not be in a hurry to "convert" family and friends to Yoga. The best way to show success is to exemplify the results. You will discover that regular practice brings on a glow from within. When people around you start noticing that you are beautiful, healthy, rested, relaxed, and happy, the message will come across by itself.

Practice Regularly and Enjoyably

As in any new endeavor, practice makes perfect. The effects of Yoga are cumulative. You will achieve the greatest—and longest-lasting—success if you make a commitment to practice some Yoga techniques every day. Set reasonable goals. Establish the length of time that is comfortable and easy for you to stick with. Then any extra time you can add on a day-to-day basis will be icing on the cake. It is a good idea also to put together a minimum routine of three or four techniques for those exceptionally busy days that come up every so often, especially if you have to travel. When traveling by plane, you can help avoid circulatory problems by practicing a few exercises. See Chapter 10 for several techniques that can be practiced on an airplane. Keeping up your Yoga practice while traveling can also help relieve symptoms of jet lag.

If, like many others, you have a tendency toward perfectionism, you may have the idea that if you don't have time to practice a full routine, there is no point in practicing at all. Not true! In Yoga even a few minutes of daily practice will do wonders for your concentration, sense of well-being, and motivation to continue happily. As a minimum, do at least three asans every day.

The time of day you practice is totally up to you. Many people find that practicing first thing in the morning gives them a wake-up boost. Others cannot spare morning time and instead practice in the late afternoon or evening. Although the practice works best if you do asans first, then breathing and meditation, you can split up the routine if necessary; for example, asans in the morning and breathing and meditation in the evening. Try to keep breathing and meditation practice together. Whatever time of day you practice, try to stick with it—even on weekends—long enough to see how well it works.

It may take several weeks to discover your own optimum routine length and the best time of day for Yoga practice, but once it is established you will find it easy to stick to it. In fact, practice will gradually become as habitual as brushing your teeth. Steady practice will pay off by carrying you through those times when it seems like you are not making much progress at all—what we call the deserts. At first the effects of Yoga practice are many and obvious, and you will experience elation at being more well and relaxed than you have ever been. After several weeks or months, however, the effects start to become more subtle; it is then that the strongest connection is made with the inner emotional-spiritual body. If you practice steadily during those times, you will be rewarded by even better, and longer-lasting, results.

Clothing

Wear clothing that is loose and/or stretchy and warm, such as loose pants with an elastic or drawstring waist, or a leotard. See Chapter 10 for techniques you can do anywhere—at the office, in line at the store—that require no change of clothing. Dress for the season, and avoid extremes of temperature in your practice room. Practice asans barefoot. When you get ready for meditation, put on a pair of socks, and have a sweater, a blanket, or something else to wrap around yourself, because your body temperature tends to drop as you relax. Your meditation experience will be best if you are warm.

Equipment

Use a blanket, mat, or large towel for exercising, even if the room is carpeted. Reserve this blanket, as well as your exercise clothing, exclusively for Yoga practice. This will help reinforce the consistency of daily practice.

If you practice seated breathing exercises on the floor, you will probably need one or more small, firm cushions. You may want to experiment with several kinds or combinations of pillows. (See the discussion of posture on p. 144.) When you lie down to meditate, you can place a pillow under your knees if you feel any discomfort in your back. Do not, however, use a pillow under the neck; doing so reduces circulation to the brain.

Environment

Try to avoid interruptions while you practice. Do not practice with pets in the room. Turn off your telephone, and put a sign on your practice room door so that you will not be disturbed. You deserve this time for yourself. With communication and patience you will be able to work out a schedule that harmonizes with your work and family responsibilities. When you are on vacation or away from your regular practice space, work out an alternate place and time for your routine. Learn to enjoy and respect privacy and silence. Avoid using music during meditation practice. Meditation is to be done in silence. Thought then springs spontaneously from your inner being.

At the office, try taking a few minutes during the day to practice some of the techniques you have learned. The breathing exercises are especially helpful. (See Chapter 10 for more suggestions.) If you do not have your own office or access to one, consider the broom closet, rest room, or supply room for a five-minute getaway. Use your coffee-break time for a brief, refreshing Yoga routine. Choose snack foods that will help you get through the day with energy: combinations of protein and carbohydrates such as yogurt and fruit, as opposed to the "empty calories" of most caffeinated beverages or sweets. For more on nutrition, see Chapter 7.

Cautions About Drugs

Never practice Yoga while under the influence of alcohol or so-called street drugs. Street drugs should be completely avoided; it is very dangerous to mix Yoga practice with drug use. Drugs disrupt normal neurological pathways to the brain; paranoia and loss of personal motivation are other common effects. I have particularly noticed this phenomenon in people who use marijuana. Although many people use drugs in order to alter consciousness, drugs also destroy concentration. Nothing could be

more devastating to the practice of Yoga. The ability to focus the mind without interruption for extended periods of time (called *ekagrata*) is one of the most valuable products of Yoga.

If you are in the habit of using drugs, even infrequently, I suggest that you abstain for a few weeks while you begin Yoga practice. You will probably find that you no longer feel the need or desire for the drugs, because you will achieve the same comforting feelings without them. The practice of Yoga techniques can supply those feelings from within.

If you are taking prescription medications, by all means follow your doctor's instructions. However, certain medications, such as large doses of tranquilizers, may affect your success with Yoga. If you are in doubt, ask your physician.

A Word About Addictions

Many authorities view addiction (the psychological and/or physical craving for something outside oneself) as a misguided response to stress. In other words, the body and mind are trying to express a need, but the body seems to be unable to supply what is needed, so we turn to mood- or mind-altering substances to help us feel better.

If you find yourself addicted to cigarettes, alcohol, sugar, caffeine, or other substances, Yoga can help. It's a healthy alternative response to stress. With Yoga you can improve your willpower, strengthen your nervous system, learn to relax at will, and better cope with the stress in your life. Give yourself a chance. Let your practice show you what it can do. Heavy smokers may experience dizziness during some exercise or breathing, as a result of their reduced lung capacity. If this is a problem for you, scale back on the number of repetitions.

Yoga and Other Forms of Exercise

People often ask me if it is beneficial to combine Yoga with other physical activities, such as running, dancing, or weight training. It is certainly a good idea to be as physically active as you can be. If you wish, you can balance the stretches of Yoga asans and relaxation training with aerobic conditioning. In Chapter 9 you will find suggestions for Yoga techniques that will help you warm up and cool down before and after sports activities.

Food and Drink

It is a good idea to wait at least 1½ hours after eating a large meal before practicing Yoga asans. If you are really hungry at practice time or it has been several hours since you ate, have a light snack (yogurt, fruit, cottage cheese, a small salad, soup, or a piece of bread) to tide you over.'

The main reason to avoid exercise immediately after eating is that a full stomach will feel very uncomfortable as you bend and compress. It will also be harder to breathe deeply. The process of digestion temporarily diverts blood flow from other areas of the body to your stomach, which is why you may feel sluggish, sleepy, or unable to concentrate well after eating. For this reason you may also find that it is harder to quiet your mind in meditation when you are full.

Because caffeine stimulates the central nervous system, it acts as a trigger for a stress response. We therefore recommend that you do not drink caffeinated beverages before practice.

Who Can Practice Yoga?

For most people, excluding those who have brilliant experience in their younger years, the ideal age to begin practice is understood to be fifty-three. It is at this time that many people in the Eastern world turn business and family matters over to their children so they can spend the rest of their lives seeking spiritual awakening.

Yoga practice was not designed for children under sixteen. Two of my great teachers, Rama and Lakshmanjoo, advised me of the danger Yoga asans pose for young children. Yoga exercises can affect the growth system, which should not be disturbed in children. For this reason, if you are under sixteen, please do not attempt the complete asan training. You can safely practice the breathing techniques, with the exception of the Kapalabhati and Agni Kriya techniques, and you can also safely practice meditation.

People these days commonly accept the fact that therapies such as acupressure and reflexology can have systemic effects from pressure applied to certain areas of the body, and the physical basis of the effect of Yoga asans may be related. The original purpose of Yoga asans was not physical culture, the way many Americans view Yoga today; instead, Yoga asans are practiced to bring the body to utmost health and strength so that the practitioner can focus on meditation and self-awareness without physical distractions. When you practice asans, you probably notice that they immediately affect your state of mind. The chemical changes in your brain begin at once, brought about by the pressure the asans put upon the body's glandular system. It's a scientific fact that brain chemistry has a direct effect on mood. Depression, for instance, is commonly corrected with Prozac or other drugs.

FINDING A YOGA TEACHER

In some ways finding a Yoga teacher is easier today than it ever was. All you have to do is go to the phone book, the Internet, or a bookstore for a list of hundreds of teachers from whom to choose. The real problem is how to know when a teacher has been adequately trained and, most important, who that person's teacher is.

As yet there is no nationally recognized standard for certification of Yoga teachers; some organizations may grant certification after attendance at a weeklong workshop; others require years of training. When you write or call to find a teacher in your area, do not be afraid to ask about qualifications; a good teacher won't mind answering your questions. What follows are a few suggestions based on our standards at the American Yoga Association.

Find out whether the teacher practices Yoga exercise, breathing, and meditation as a daily discipline or just occasionally as one of a number of other activities. Does the teacher study regularly with a teacher of his or her own? This is important, because Yoga is a continual learning process. The need for a teacher never disappears. American Yoga Association teachers are all committed to daily practice and undergo a constant review of their practice with me.

A genuine teacher lives a genuine Yogic lifestyle. The ethic of Nonviolence demands that teachers be vegetarian, because violence can be transferred in class when there is an acceptance of killing for food. Teachers do not smoke or use street drugs. Their conduct is responsible, safe, and aware, based on the ethical guidelines set forth by Patanjali. (See Chapter 11 for more on Yoga philosophy, as well as my book *Yoga of the Heart* for a complete discussion of ethics in Yoga.)

A good Yoga teacher is strictly ethical and has spent time studying the various effects of Yoga exercises, breathing, and meditation. She or he has a working knowledge of major muscle groups and body systems, and is able to vary the techniques according to each person's capability. Yoga is not a religion, and a genuine Yoga teacher will not infuse the Yoga techniques with his or her own religious beliefs.

These guidelines may seem strict, but the American Yoga Association believes that teachers of Yoga must be exceptionally conscientious and professional in their work of teaching the exacting discipline of Yoga. These personal commitments ensure that teachers will avoid any injury or misrepresentation in their classes and allow them to teach Yoga in an educational, nonreligious format to students of every background. Individuals have a right to choose the religion they wish to follow without being influenced by others.

HOW TO PRACTICE YOGA ASANS

Before beginning practice, read all of this chapter and heed the cautionary notes. Again, check with your doctor before starting any new exercise program.

Always Warm Up

Always warm up before starting a routine. If your time is limited, do the first half of the warm-up routine only (through the Lazy Stretch exercise).

Follow Curriculum and Instructions

The American Yoga Association suggests that Yoga is best approached in a holistic manner, with a complete program of ethics, exercise, breathing, and meditation. In the next chapter you will read about warming up. Chapter 2 describes a complete routine that should be followed by every student of Yoga, regardless of level of proficiency. Following that, we outline a curriculum of three courses, each ten weeks in length, approximating the format of the classes we teach. For best results, follow the curriculum as outlined and include some exercise, breathing, and meditation in each practice session. You can cut down on your total practice time if you have a busy schedule, or split your daily practice into two sessions if necessary. To help you remember which exercises go with which course, each exercise in Chapter 3 is marked for Course 1, 2, and/or 3.

When you have warmed up and are ready to start the asans, read the instructions and then try the exercises, following the illustrations. Keep this book alongside your mat for reference. Reread the instructions to make sure you are following them correctly. Especially note the breath instructions with each exercise. Correct breathing will help improve the efficacy of your exercise. Repeat each exercise as directed.

To increase your focus when practicing Yoga asans, count to three silently with each section of the exercise and during the momentary holds. This practice will help you concentrate and encourage fluid movements. Each exercise includes specific instructions on how to add this feature. Count as slowly or quickly as you need to to avoid getting winded.

Breathe Deeply and Slowly

In most exercises you will be instructed to breathe deeply and slowly along with the three-count just described. Do not hold your breath except when specified. At no time should you hold your breath for more than 5 seconds.

Always breathe in and out through your nose while exercising, unless your physician has specifically advised you to breathe out through your mouth. Breathing through the nose helps you maintain control over the length and smoothness of your breath and speeds the efficacy of practice.

Move Slowly and Deliberately

Concentrate on making slow, careful, and smooth movements. Remember that the process of moving through an exercise is just as important as the goal—attaining a particular position. Never bounce, jerk, or bend quickly. Yoga stretches and strengthens delicate nerve and muscle tissues, so move slowly and gently. Be aware of areas of strain or tension. Respect them. At times you will be instructed to hold positions while breathing gently. This hold greatly increases the effectiveness of the exercise.

Repetitions

Except for the warm-up sequence, Yoga asans are to be repeated three times each. We recommend that you practice your routine daily. Practicing asan routines more than once a day may overstimulate your nervous system, making you tense, irritable, or high-strung. If you want to exercise at another time of day, do some aerobic conditioning instead.

Rest Periodically

After every three or four asans, rest for a minute or so. Completely relax; let yourself go limp. I tell my students to imagine themselves as a piece of wet liver. Try to stop all thought; let your mind and body rest.

Allow for Variations in Balance and Limberness

Because your body is greatly affected by your reaction to stress, how well you sleep, your diet, and many other factors, you will find that your limberness and sense of balance will vary from day to day. Everyone is slightly stiff in the morning. Do not be discouraged by these slight variations; if you practice daily, you will notice a steady overall progression. The important thing is not how well you perform your asans on a particular day but rather that you do them every day.

Do Not Exercise When Ill

Do not exercise when you are ill, even if it's "just a cold." No matter how mild the illness, your body needs rest more than anything else, not for you to make additional demands on it. In some instances, such as with a sinus infection or head cold, exercising may even spread the infection or at least aggravate your symptoms. You *can* practice breathing and meditation techniques at any time.

Special Notes for Women

We strongly advise you not to practice strenuous Yoga asans during your menstrual period. Many Yoga asans impose pressure on and stretch the abdominal area, and this can cause increased bleeding. Yoga exercises stimulate your hormonal system and, combined with the natural hormonal changes of your period, may lead to increased nervousness, irritability, or upset. Take a break from asans during your period, and use the extra time for meditation and study.

NURSING MOTHERS
We suggest that nursing mothers refrain from Yoga asans until their babies have been completely weaned. We believe that the hormonal changes brought about by Yoga asans are evident in the chemical composition of the mother's milk and are not suitable for the well-being of the child. Meditation and breath exercises are encouraged and may be practiced any time.

PREGNANCY
If you are pregnant, we recommend that you do no asans at all during the first trimester. After that you may practice a limited routine if there have been no complications and your physician approves (see Chapter 8). You may find that practice of certain Yoga asans during the last six months of your term results in an easier delivery and a more relaxed, happier baby. If you decide to take Lamaze classes, you will find that Yoga harmonizes with those techniques very well. Meditation and simple breathing exercises may be safely practiced during your entire pregnancy.

Chapter 2

GETTING READY TO EXERCISE: THE YOGA WARM-UP

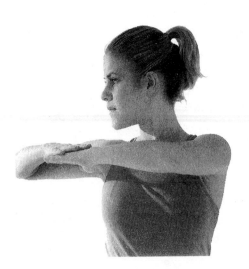

*N*ow you are ready to begin practicing Yoga. First comes a proper warm-up. Before you start, make sure you have read Chapter 1 thoroughly and understand all the cautions and suggestions. A complete curriculum for three ten-week courses is outlined in Chapter 3.

In the weekly curriculum lists, the warm-up exercises are listed not separately but as a group: the Warm-up Sequence. After a few weeks of practice you'll know the warm-ups so well that you will not have to refer back to the instructions in this chapter.

Whether you are a rank beginner or have practiced for several years, it is best to warm up before every session, using the sequence in this chapter. Warming up has nothing to do with the temperature of the room or how limber your body may already feel. Yoga exercises work not only the large muscle groups but also delicate nerves, connective tissue, blood vessels, and internal organs. Warming up prepares your whole body for exercise, so that it begins easily and without a lot of fear or tension. The body is often afraid to start a new discipline. If you are rushed or especially tense, you may want to spend extra time warming up or even use the Warm-up Sequence as your entire exercise commitment for the day.

Warming up is also an opportunity to warm up—or rather, relax—your mind, quieting extraneous thoughts and centering yourself.

As you warm up, pay attention to what your body is saying to you. Is it expressing tension or pain anywhere? Is it fatigued, strained, ill, or angry? Learn to listen for your body's signals;

you'll discover more about how your body works, how it reacts, and what it needs. Do this in silence. Remember what you observed as you begin to do more vigorous exercises. Your body will resist growth with pain if it is forced or bullied; a gentle approach yields positive changes much more quickly. There is no need for self-violence.

Shoulder Rolls

- Limber shoulder joints
- Reduce tension in upper back and neck muscles
- Improve posture
- Can help relieve arthritic stiffness and pain in shoulder joints

Stand with arms at your sides. Let them hang loose like wet spaghetti (A). Lift both shoulders up toward your ears (B), then roll them in a circle forward (C), down, back (D), and up toward your ears again. Repeat in the opposite direction. Repetitions: 3 to 5 each direction. Breathe normally; don't hold your breath. To help loosen and relax especially stiff shoulders, massage your shoulders and neck before and after this exercise. Shake out your arms afterwards to relax them.

Keep your arms and hands limp.
Breathe normally.

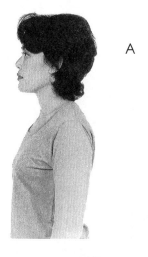

A

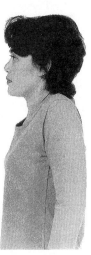

B

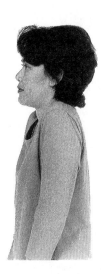

C

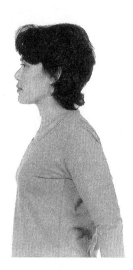

D

Elbow Touch

- Limbers shoulder joints
- Reduces tension in upper and mid-back muscle groups
- Improves posture

Bring your fingertips to your shoulders, with your elbows raised shoulder-high. Slowly bring your elbows together in front (A), then apart to the sides and back (B), squeezing your shoulder blades together. Breathe normally. Don't hold your breath. Repetitions: 3 to 5.

Breathe normally.
Keep your upper arms and elbows horizontal to the floor.

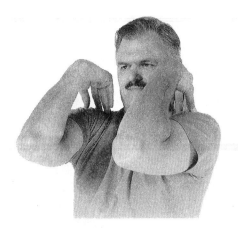

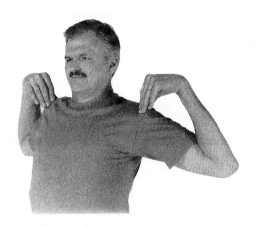

A   B

Arm Rolls

- Limber shoulder joints
- Stretch and strengthen upper back muscles
- Stimulate nerves in arms
- Improve circulation in torso, neck, and head

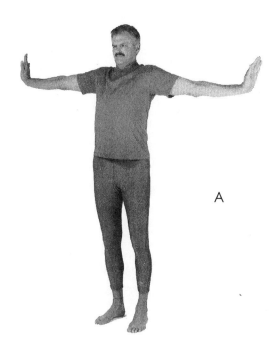

A

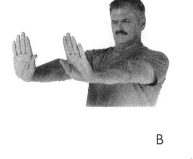

B

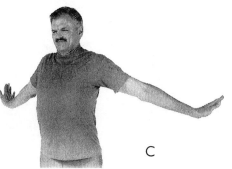

C

Raise arms straight out to the sides, holding them parallel to the floor. Flex your hands back, as if stopping traffic to your left and right (A). Now rotate your arms forward in large circles, first bringing your hands almost together in front (B), then rotating as far back as your shoulder joints will allow (C). Move slowly. Breathe normally. Repetitions: 3 to 5 circles in each direction. Keep your fingers flexed during the entire movement, and your elbows straight.

Relax your arms to the sides and shake out shoulders, arms, and lower back, relaxing the muscles and nerves.

Continue with smaller, faster circles, about the size of a dinner plate. Remember to do the same number of circles in both directions.

Note: If you have high blood pressure or heart disease (and your doctor's permission to practice Yoga), do not attempt the smaller rotations—which put extra strain on the heart muscles—until you have practiced the large ones for several months. The extra circulation brought about by this exercise will make your upper body feel warm and flushed. Check with your doctor if you have any doubts about whether to practice this variation.

Keep your fingers flexed and elbows straight.
Breathe normally.
Make large circles as big as possible, small
 ones the size of dinner plates.

Neck Stretch

- Limbers neck and improves circulation through-out neck region
- Reduces tension in neck muscles
- Limbers cervical spine

There are several options for arm positions in this exercise. We recommend that you start with straight arms extended to the sides, palms up (A). If this causes fatigue, you can rest your hands on your hips or let them hang at your sides. Choose the position that best helps you keep your shoulders from tensing or lifting as you move your head. This stretch is intended to exercise the neck muscles only; the rest of your body should remain relaxed.

Start by lowering your chin to your chest (B); then lift your chin so you are looking up at the ceiling (C). (Avoid dropping your head all the way back because of the extra strain this causes on the neck.) Repetitions: 3, breathing normally.

Next, start with your head straight, tilt your head to the right, ear over your shoulder (D), then lift your head and gently tilt to the left (E). Try not to lift your shoulder up toward your ear; move only the head. Breathe normally. Repetitions: 3.

Now, from the start position (A), turn your head to the right and look over your right shoulder (F), then turn to the left (G). Repetitions: 3.

Note: If you have a neck injury or pain or stiffness in your neck, stop here. If not, go on to the final two variations.

Variation: This variation moves your neck in a gentle semicircle back and forth. Start by lowering your chin to your chest (B). Slowly roll your head to the right until you reach the right "tilt" position: ear over your right shoulder (D). Roll your head back down to your chest (B) and over to your left (E). Continue the back-and-forth movement for a total of 3 right-to-left-to-right repetitions.

Variation: If the previous variation gives your neck no problem, go on to this variation: Starting with your chin lowered to your chest (B), slowly rotate your head to the right, ear over your shoulder (D), remembering to keep shoulders relaxed throughout; then roll your head up and over to your left shoulder (E), and finally roll your head forward to the start position. Relax your arms and shake them out. Repetitions: 3 in each direction.

Keep your mouth closed, lips together.
Breathe normally.
Do not lift your shoulders.
Move slowly.
Do not drop the head back too far.

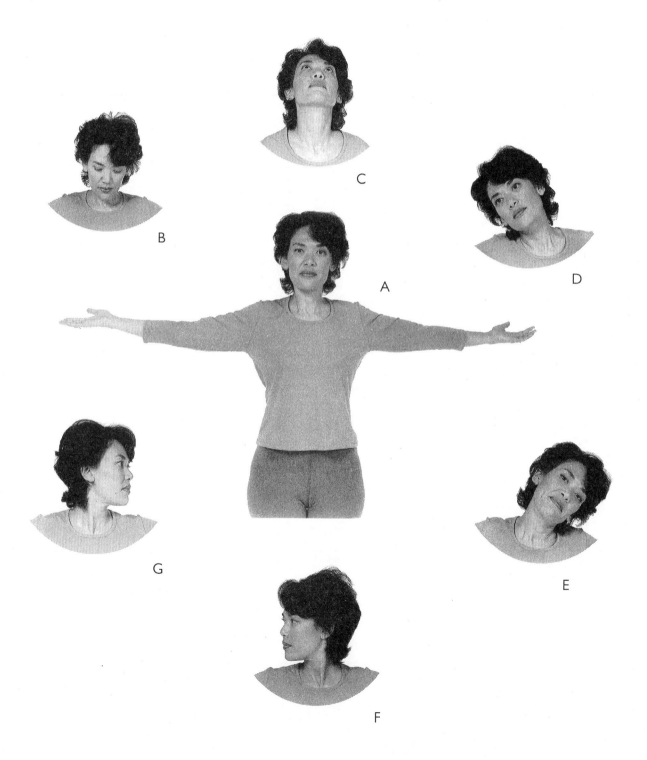

Standing Reach

- Limbers and strengthens shoulder joints
- Expands rib cage
- Strengthens ankles and calves
- Improves balance

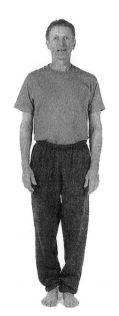

A

Stand with your arms relaxed at your sides, and breathe out completely (A). Fix your gaze on a spot on the floor or wall; this will help you keep your balance. Breathe in and count to three as you raise your arms in a wide circle to the sides, then overhead as you come up on your toes (B). Hold your breath for a count of three as you press your palms together and stretch a little farther up, toward the ceiling. Breathe out for a count of three as you lower your arms to the sides and down, and your heels to the floor. Repetitions: 3.

On days when your balance is less steady, divide this exercise in two, using the same three-count breath: first, breathe in and lift your arms out to the sides and up overhead. Press your palms together and stretch, then breathe out as you lower your arms out and down. Next, holding on to a chair or bar for balance, breathe in to a count of three as you come up on your toes, then breathe out and lower your heels to the floor. Repetitions: 3 for each part.

Stare at one spot for balance.
Breathe deeply through your nose.

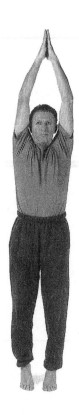

B

Easy Bend

- Limbers upper back muscles and shoulder joints
- Improves circulation to head
- Relieves tension in upper back and neck
- Gives a light stretch to muscles and nerves in legs, back, and neck

Stand straight with feet parallel, arms relaxed at your sides (A). Breathe out. Now breathe in and count to three as you raise your arms to the sides until they are parallel to the floor, palms facing front (B). Hold for a count of three. Now breathe out and count to three as you bend forward, head first, pulling out of your hips. Picture yourself diving for the correct stretch. Let your head and arms relax completely (C). Bend only halfway (even if you can easily bend much farther), so that your hands hang at about the level of your knees. Breathe in as you straighten up, raising your arms again to the sides.

Repeat, breathing out to a count of three as you bend forward and breathing in as you straighten up. Try to match your breath to your movement so that your exhalation lasts for the whole movement down and forward and your inhalation lasts for the whole movement back up. Repetitions: 3. After the last inhalation, breathe out to a count of three and relax, slowly lowering your arms to the sides to the start position (A).

Breathe through your nose.
Try to match your breath to your movement.
Relax your head, neck, arms, and hands completely in the forward position.
Move slowly and deliberately—but not so slowly that you start gasping for breath.

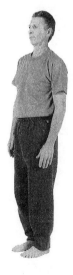

A

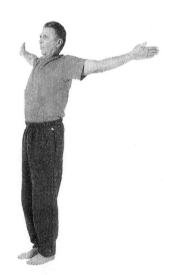

B

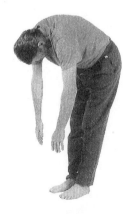

C

Lazy Stretch

- Stretches backs of legs
- Begins to limber lower back

With your feet parallel and a few inches apart, bend your knees slightly. Rest your forearms on your knees and clasp your hands together. Lift your head slightly and breathe in to a count of three (A). Hold for a count of three. Now breathe out to a count of three as you tuck your head and straighten your legs as much as possible, keeping your elbows in place (B). Repetitions: 3 to 5.

Coordinate breath and movement.
Don't stretch to the point of discomfort.
Remember to lift the head on inhalation and
     tuck the head on exhalation.

Full Bend

- Stretches nerves and muscles along backs of legs and spine all the way up to back of head, which may help sciatic nerve problems and varicose veins
- Improves circulation to entire body
- Strengthens respiratory and heart muscles
- Strengthens postural muscles
- Strengthens lower back

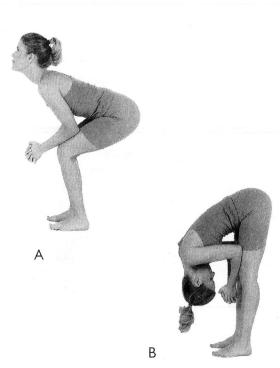

A

B

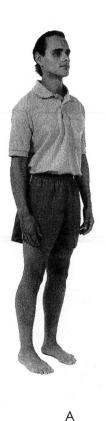

A

Start with your feet parallel, arms at your sides (A). Breathe in and count to three as you bring your arms up and out to the sides, expanding your chest (B). Hold your breath for a count of three, then breathe out (through your nose, remember) as you count to three, bending forward from the hips (C). As you bend, reach your arms down, toward the floor. Rest them in front of your feet, if possible. When you have bent forward as far as you can, your exhalation should be complete. Make sure your neck, head, arms, and hands are limp at this point (D). Now start to breathe in and slowly straighten, bringing your arms up and out to the sides as before. Your head comes up last. As you become more limber, try stretching a little farther, until your hands reach the floor.

Repeat this rhythmic up-and-down motion, counting to three with each movement: arms up, hold, down, lift. Try to match your breath to your movement. Move slowly, but not so slowly that you start gasping for breath. Usually, beginners can comfortably complete each movement in 3 to 5 seconds. Repetitions: 3 to 5.

Coordinate breath with movement.
Move slowly and deliberately.
Don't strain to reach the floor.
Breathe through your nose.

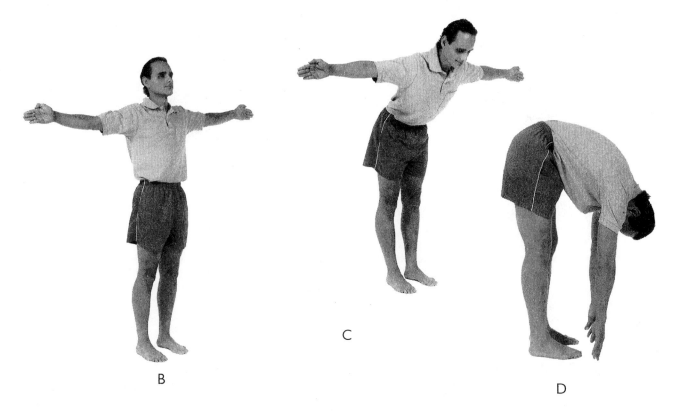

B

C

D

Elbow Twist

- Improves flexibility in spinal column
- Relieves tension in upper back and shoulders

Stand with your feet parallel, a few inches apart. Lift your arms in front of you, elbows bent, placing one hand on top of the other (A). Twist slowly to the right (B), then to the left (C), leading with your elbows. After a couple of cycles, add the following

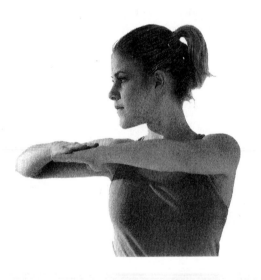

B

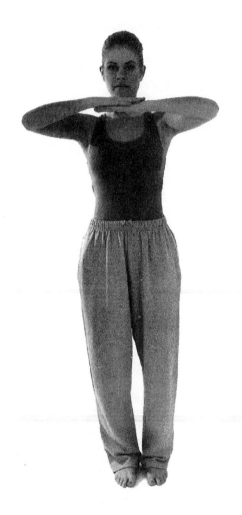

A

breath pattern: Breathe out as you twist to the side, breathe in as you return to the front, breathe out to the other side, breathe in to the front, and so on. Count to three with each movement. Keep your arms parallel to the floor, back straight. Concentrate on the gentle twisting motion of your spine. Repetitions: 3 to 5 in each direction.

Your head should turn with your body so that there is no extra twist to the neck. For a variation, however, you can turn your head and arms in opposite directions. (Do not do this variation if you have chronic pain or stiffness in your neck.) Another variation is to begin with arms overhead, lowering them to your waist as you twist.

Breathe out as you twist to the side, and
    breathe in going back to the front.
Keep the rest of your body (especially your
    stomach!) relaxed.
Try to twist from the hips rather than from the
    knees.

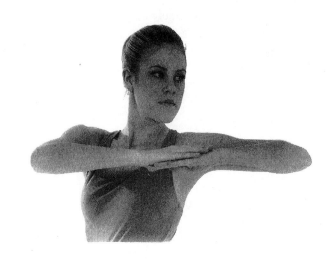

C

Leg Lifts

- Strengthen and tone leg muscles
- Improve balance
- Stretch backs of legs
- Improve circulation in legs and lower torso

Raise arms straight out in front of you, palms down. Breathe in for a count of three as you lift your straight right leg toward your hands, toes flexed (A). This is a controlled lift, not a kick. Breathe out for a count of three as you lower the leg. Keeping your knees straight is much more important than touching your toes to your hands. Repeat with the left leg. Repetitions: 3 to 5 each leg.

On days when your balance is shaky, hold on to the back of a chair with one hand and extend the other.

Now extend both arms out to the sides and breathe in for a count of three as you lift your right leg to the side (B). Instead of "turning out" your leg, as you would in a ballet class (so that your knee and toes point to the ceiling), keep your knee and flexed foot pointed forward so that you will lift and strengthen the muscles and nerves along the sides of your hip and leg. Breathe out for a count of three as you lower the leg. Repeat with the left leg. Repetitions: 3 to 5 each leg.

Then, with both arms extended to the back, palms facing each other, breathe in for a count of three as

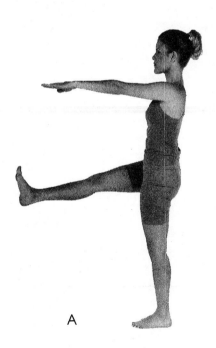

A

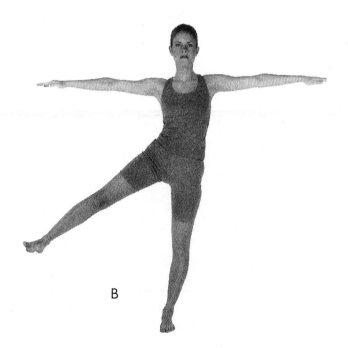

B

you slowly lift your left leg backward, keeping it straight (C). Breathe out to a count of three as you lower the leg. Do not lean forward; instead, use the muscles in your back and buttock to lift the leg. Try not to bend your knee as you lift. Repetitions: 3 to 5 each leg.

> Keep your legs straight and toes flexed at all times.
> Keep your torso straight.

Complete Leg Lifts: Variation

- Strengthen hip joints and lower back
- Improve balance
- Strengthen nerves and tone muscles in legs and hips
- Reduce body fat

Standing with both hands on your hips, stare at one spot for balance. Breathe in to a count of three as you slowly raise your right leg to the front, keeping your toes flexed and knees straight. Keeping your foot raised and your breath held in, slowly move your leg out to the side, toes pointed forward, then to the back, trying not to lean forward to compensate. Breathe out to a count of three as you return your foot to the floor. Still using the right leg and continuing the three-count, reverse direction, lifting your leg first to the back, then to the side, then to the front. Repeat with the left leg.

> Keep your foot flexed.
> Keep your legs straight.
> Keep your torso erect.

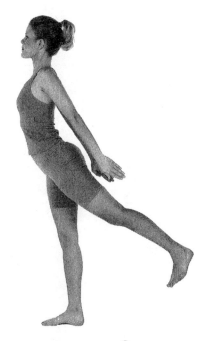

C

Standing Knee Squeeze

- May improve digestive function
- Limbers hip joints and knees
- Strengthens back and legs
- Improves balance and circulation
- Helps relieve lower back tension

Stand with feet parallel. Breathe out. Now breathe in and count to three as you raise your left knee and grasp it with both hands. Hold your breath in for a count of three as you squeeze the knee toward your body (A). Remember to stare at one spot for balance. Relax your foot rather than flexing it. Breathe out as you count to three and lower your foot to the floor. Repeat with your right knee.

After a few days, add this variation: After releasing your knee, reach behind you to grasp the ankle of the same leg and squeeze the leg to the back while exhaling with your three-count (B).

Variation: If you have arthritis in your knees or an injury that makes squeezing your knee painful, grasp your thigh instead. You will feel the same compression on your stomach without straining your knee. Repetitions: 3 each leg, alternating.

On days when your balance is less steady, hold on to a chair back with one hand and squeeze the lifted knee with the other (C), or lean your back or side against a wall.

Stare at one spot.
Hold your breath in while squeezing the knee.
Relax your foot.

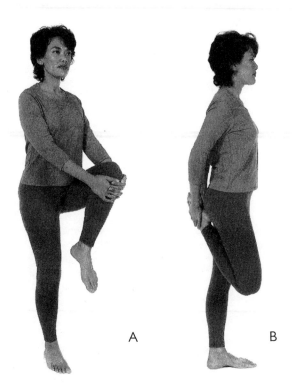

A   B

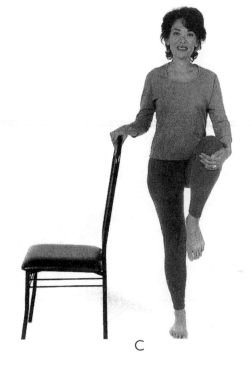

C

Massage Knees and Ankles

● Warms and relaxes knee and ankle joints

Sit on the floor with your legs extended in front of you. Massage each knee (A) and ankle (B) for several seconds with both hands. Rub lightly, using your whole hands, until the joint feels warm.

Note: Rubbing your joints regularly with oil or lotion will help them limber up more quickly.

Rotate each ankle several times clockwise, then counterclockwise.
Use your whole hands when massaging—not just your fingers.

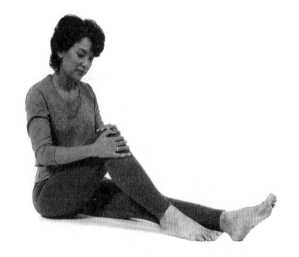

A

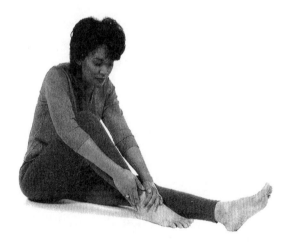

B

Hands and Knees Stretch

- Limbers lower back
- Stretches chest muscles
- Loosens hip and knee joints

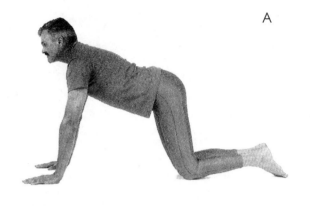

A

Sitting on your feet on the floor, breathe out. Then breathe in and count to three as you come forward so that you are on all fours (A). Then gently drop your hips forward and down as you look up. Keep your arms stiff (B). Breathe out and count to three as you sit back on your feet. Your arms stay out in front, and your head falls forward between them (C). Repetitions: 3 to 5.

Keep your arms straight.
Look up on inhalation.

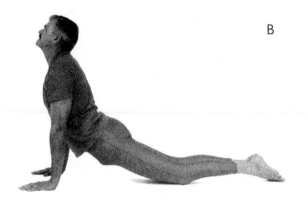

B

Note: If you have trouble sitting on your feet because of knee or ankle problems, begin on all fours and rock back on the exhalation as far as you can without strain.

If you have neck or upper back problems, do not tilt your head back as shown; instead, keep looking straight ahead.

Hands and Knees Stretch with Double Breath

(Course 3 only)

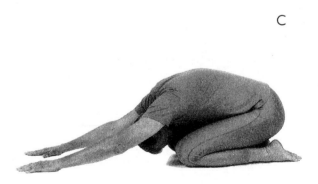

C

In the first two versions of the Emotional Stability Routine introduced in Course 3, this exercise is performed a bit faster, and the breath pattern changes as follows: Breathe out in the extreme forward and back positions and breathe in between, so that each complete repetition includes two inhalations and two exhalations.

Chapter 3

PUTTING IT ALL TOGETHER: CURRICULUM AND ROUTINES

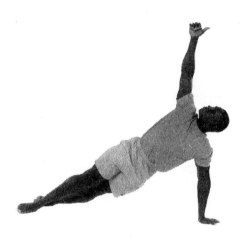

The courses and special routines outlined in this chapter are based on our current beginner's curriculum of three consecutive ten-week courses. You may find you progress slightly slower or faster, since each of us has unique strengths and goals. The important thing is that you don't become so eager to progress that you strain yourself or push on to a more advanced program before you are comfortable with each technique. The Maintenance Routines at the end of each section are designed to help you practice the fine points until you feel ready to go on to the next course. Asterisks indicate techniques new to that particular week or course.

It's helpful to understand how the techniques fit together. We feel that Yoga is approached best as a balanced experience encompassing exercise, breathing, and meditation, and our classes include some of each of these elements each week. If you don't have a lot of time to spend on Yoga each day, you will maximize the benefits by including the three elements in your daily practice session. At a minimum, practice three exercises daily.

You will find all the exercises described and illustrated in Chapter 4: Exercise *(Asana)*. Breathing and meditation are described in Chapters 5 and 6. The Warm-up Sequence is the same for each course. Warming up is so important that it has been given its own chapter. If you have skipped the previous chapter, go back and read it now.

In Chapter 4 the Yoga exercises are presented in a progression from standing to kneeling to sitting and finally prone. We have organized the exercises this way so that you do not have to flip back and forth in the book as you follow the curriculum. You will notice that each exercise is marked as Course 1, 2, and/or 3. Advanced exercises are shown alongside their simpler versions. *Please do not attempt the more advanced version until the curriculum instructs you to do so.* That way, you will avoid injury or stress by building your flexibility, strength, and stamina gradually and safely.

As you follow the course guidelines, remember the importance of making a smooth transition from one exercise to the next. Many students ask if the techniques should be done in sequence as listed, with the exercises first, then the breathing, then the meditation. Practicing the asans and breathing first helps to prepare the mind for meditation; however, if you cannot spare time for an entire routine all at once, you may practice asans at one time of day and breathing and meditation at another.

COURSE ONE

Introduction

Remember that the following routines are suggestions only. If you find the pace difficult, take two weeks or longer to practice each routine before moving on. If the routine is very easy for you and you have extra time, add one or two new exercises each week so that you move along a little more quickly. During the first month, practice the exercises for the recommended amount of time and in the order in which they are given. In each course the sequence of asans is designed so that you can move easily from one to the next, and from standing to kneeling to sitting, and finally to lying down.

Here are the objectives for the first ten weeks of a Yoga program:

1. Strengthen and stretch the spine and legs
2. Improve circulation
3. Begin to limber the hips and knee joints
4. Learn to coordinate the breath with the asans
5. Improve your kinesthetic sense
6. Improve balance and coordination
7. Stretch major muscle groups
8. Begin to communicate with your body
9. Improve respiration and oxygenation
10. Learn to breathe correctly and completely
11. Practice using the breath to reduce stress reactions
12. Stretch and strengthen the breathing musculature
13. Practice extension and control of the breath
14. Refresh and recharge your mind
15. Learn to relax at will
16. Recognize and release muscle tension
17. Practice observation of sensory input and other mental activities
18. Recognize emotional stress reactions
19. Improve concentration

The most important goal in the first few weeks is to find the best way to fit your Yoga practice into your daily schedule. Try not to set impossible goals. Start with a modest time commitment—as little as 5 minutes will do—that you know you can achieve every single day, even if you have a hectic schedule. Think of times during the day when you can fit in a technique or two (see Chapter 10 for ideas). Then any additional time you can devote to your practice will be a bonus. You will feel better about yourself when you can fulfill your commitment and keep your word to yourself. That feeling will motivate you to continue practicing.

WEEKLY CURRICULUM

(*Indicates new exercise)

WEEK ONE

ASANS

Warm-up Sequence (p. 24)

Easy Balance (p. 64)

Stretching Dog (p. 66)

Alternate Triangle (p. 69)

Corpse Pose Rest (p. 63)

Knee Squeeze (single only) (p. 113)

Foot Flaps (p. 99)

Seated Sun Pose (p. 100)

Baby Pose (p. 84)

Back Strengtheners (single arm and alternate arm
   and leg only) (p. 130)

BREATHING (Breath Warm-ups)

Back Arch (p. 146)

Arm Swing (p. 147)

Arm Reach (p. 148)

Belly Breath (10 repetitions or more per day to
   start) (p. 149)

MEDITATION

10 to 15 minutes, lying down

WEEK TWO

ASANS

Warm-up Sequence

Easy Balance

Stretching Dog

Alternate Triangle

*Standing Sun Pose (p. 82)

Corpse Pose Rest

Knee Squeeze (*add double) (p. 113)

Foot Flaps

Seated Sun Pose

Baby Pose

Back Strengtheners (*add arms only and legs only)
   (p. 130)

BREATHING

All Breath Warm-ups

*Complete Breath (p. 150)

MEDITATION

10 to 15 minutes

WEEK THREE

ASANS

Warm-up Sequence

Easy Balance

Stretching Dog

Alternate Triangle

Standing Sun Pose

Corpse Pose Rest

Knee Squeeze

Foot Flaps

Seated Sun Pose

*Alternate Seated Sun Pose (p. 103)

Baby Pose

Back Strengtheners

*Boat Pose (p. 132)

BREATHING

All Breath Warm-ups

*Lion (p. 153)

Complete Breath; work on rhythm and smoothness

MEDITATION

10 to 15 minutes

*Body Talk (p. 44)

WEEK FOUR

ASANS

Warm-up Sequence

Easy Balance

*Easy Balance Twist (p. 65)

*Complete Leg Lifts (p. 37)

Stretching Dog

Alternate Triangle

Standing Sun Pose

Corpse Pose Rest

Knee Squeeze

Foot Flaps

Seated Sun Pose

Alternate Seated Sun Pose

Baby Pose

*Easy Cobra Pose (p. 136)

Back Strengtheners

Boat Pose

BREATHING

All Breath Warm-ups

Lion

Complete Breath; start timing your breath using a clock (p. 151); start using earplugs (p. 152)

MEDITATION

10 to 15 minutes

In the third week, we insert the following exercise to augment communication with your body. After you have been practicing the techniques for a couple of weeks and have had a chance to observe how they are affecting you, try this exercise.

Body Talk

Have you ever noticed how difficult it is to think creatively when you are ill or injured? When you are immersed in an emotional or intellectual problem, do you find yourself resistant to devoting attention to taking care of your body? The mind and body are intimately connected; anything you do to one will automatically affect the other.

Try having a conversation with your body to find out more about its needs. Have paper and pen ready. Sit in a comfortable position, close your eyes, and for a few minutes think about your relationship with your body. Has it changed over time? Try to remember as many physical experiences as you can, and make a list of them. Include some from childhood and adolescence, as well as more current experiences. Some examples: learning to ride a bike, scoring a touchdown for your high school football team, giving birth, playing on the company softball team.

Now try to remember how you felt about your body at each of these moments. For example, everyone goes through dramatic physical changes in early adolescence. Try to remember how you felt about your body—its look, shape, and capabilities—during that period of your life.

Now just relax, close your eyes, and take a few deep breaths. Try to quiet your mind. When you feel relaxed, open your eyes and write down a greeting to your body. Imagine that you are standing in front of a mirror and that your body can speak to you. What would it say? Write down whatever comes into your mind. Now close your eyes again, relax, quiet your mind, breathe deeply, and wait until a response to what your body has said occurs to you. Write that down. Continue the conversation with your body, back and forth. If you have a physical problem, ask your body specifically about that problem.

At the end of 10 minutes or so you should have a brief written conversation that may tell you something about your body's feelings, needs, and desires. Even if it seems as if you are making up the whole conversation, your imagination is largely fueled by your unconscious, and you may be surprised by what your body has to say.

Normally we listen to our bodies only when they send us signals that are loud and clear. They tell us when we're in pain or straining, hungry, thirsty, or exhausted. By regularly tuning in to your body with this technique, you will gradually develop a much healthier relationship with it. You'll learn to recognize its warning signals so that you can relax muscle tension before it develops into a headache or stomach upset. Your body can even tell you the kinds of food it most needs. You will also grow to respect the amazing ways your body functions in order to maintain the precious gift of life that allows us to grow and learn.

WEEK FIVE

ASANS

Warm-up Sequence
Easy Balance
Easy Balance Twist
Complete Leg Lifts
Stretching Dog
Alternate Triangle
*Full Triangle (p. 68)
Standing Sun Pose
Corpse Pose Rest
Knee Squeeze
Foot Flaps
Seated Sun Pose
Alternate Seated Sun Pose
Baby Pose
Easy and *Regular Cobra Poses (p. 137)
Back Strengtheners

Boat Pose
*Easy Bridge (p. 119)
BREATHING
All Breath Warm-ups
Lion
Complete Breath; continue timing breath
MEDITATION
10 to 15 minutes

WEEK SIX

ASANS

Warm-up Sequence
Easy Balance and Twist
Complete Leg Lifts
*Tree Pose (p. 74)
Stretching Dog
Alternate Triangle
Standing Sun Pose
Corpse Pose Rest
Knee Squeeze
Foot Flaps
Seated Sun Pose
Alternate Seated Sun Pose
*Limber Hips (p. 104)
Baby Pose
*Easy Spine Twist (p. 105)
Back Strengtheners
Boat Pose
*The Roll (p. 123)
Easy Bridge
BREATHING
All Breath Warm-ups
Lion
Complete Breath
*Humming Breath (p. 152)

MEDITATION

10 to 15 minutes

By this time you have added so many new asans to your repertoire that, unless you can devote more and more time to practice, you'll have trouble fitting everything in. Don't despair. Instead, each day skip several of the earlier asans, but alternate the ones you skip so you continue to practice each. Alternatively, you may use the shorter routines on pp. 48 and 49 when time is limited.

WEEK SEVEN

ASANS

Warm-up Sequence

Easy Balance and Twist

Complete Leg Lifts

Tree Pose

*Dancer Pose (p. 76)

Stretching Dog

Alternate Triangle

Full Triangle

Standing Sun Pose

Corpse Pose Rest

Knee Squeeze

Foot Flaps

Seated Sun Pose

Alternate Seated Sun Pose

Limber Hips

Baby Pose

*Spine Twist (p. 106)

*Diamond Pose Warm-up (p. 108)

*Diamond Pose (p. 109)

Boat Pose

*Bow Pose (p. 138)

The Roll

Easy Bridge

BREATHING

All Breath Warm-ups

Lion

Complete Breath; continue timing breath occasionally

Humming Breath

MEDITATION

10 to 15 minutes

WEEK EIGHT

ASANS

Warm-up Sequence

Easy Balance and Twist

Complete Leg Lifts

Tree Pose

Stretching Dog

Alternate Triangle

Full Triangle

Standing Sun Pose

Corpse Pose Rest

Knee Squeeze

Foot Flaps

Seated Sun Pose

Alternate Seated Sun Pose

Limber Hips

Baby Pose

*Arm and Leg Balance (p. 86)

*Bow Variation (p. 89)

Spine Twist

Bow Pose

Boat Pose

The Roll

*Shoulder Stand (p. 124)

Easy Bridge

BREATHING

All Breath Warm-ups

Lion

Complete Breath; continue timing breath
    occasionally

Humming Breath

MEDITATION

    15 to 20 minutes

WEEK NINE

ASANS

    Warm-up Sequence

    Easy Balance and Twist

    Complete Leg Lifts

    Tree Pose

    Dancer Pose

    *T Pose (p. 78)

    *Standing Rest (p. 63)

    Stretching Dog

    Alternate Triangle

    Full Triangle

    Standing Sun Pose

    Corpse Pose Rest

    Knee Squeeze

    Foot Flaps

    Seated Sun Pose

    Alternate Seated Sun Pose

    Limber Hips

    Baby Pose

    Alternate Arm and Leg Balance

    Bow Variation

    *Cat Breath (p. 87)

    Spine Twist

    Back Strengtheners

    Boat Pose

    The Roll

    Shoulder Stand

    *Pelvic Twist (p. 118)

    *Intense Floor Stretch (p. 112)

    Easy Bridge

BREATHING

    All Breath Warm-ups

    Lion

    Complete Breath

    Humming Breath

MEDITATION

    15 to 20 minutes

WEEK TEN

ASANS

    Warm-up Sequence

    Easy Balance and Twist

    Complete Leg Lifts

    Tree Pose

    Dancer Pose

    T Pose

    Standing Rest

    Stretching Dog

    Alternate Triangle

    Full Triangle

    Standing Sun Pose

    Corpse Pose Rest

    Knee Squeeze

    Foot Flaps

    Seated Sun Pose

    Alternate Seated Sun Pose

    Limber Hips

    Baby Pose

    Alternate Arm and Leg Balance

    Bow Variation

    Cat Breath

    Spine Twist

    Back Strengtheners

    Boat Pose

    The Roll

    Shoulder Stand

    *Plow Pose (p. 126)

Pelvic Twist
Intense Floor Stretch
Easy Bridge
BREATHING
All Breath Warm-ups
Lion
Complete Breath
Humming Breath
MEDITATION
15 to 20 minutes

FATIGUE-REDUCING ROUTINE

Try this shorter routine on days when you are tired and don't have time for a full asan routine. Asans that compress (such as the Knee Squeezes) or those that bend backward (such as the Easy Cobra) are the most effective stress relievers, because they help relax tensed breathing and release tight postural muscles.

SHOULDER ROLLS, p. 25

ELBOW TOUCH, p. 26

EASY BEND, THEN HANG HEAD DOWN FOR
    SEVERAL SECONDS, p. 31

EASY BALANCE, p. 64

BABY POSE, p. 84

CAT BREATH, p. 87

EASY COBRA POSE, p. 136

EASY SPINE TWIST, p. 105

KNEE SQUEEZE, p. 113

EASY BRIDGE, p. 119

Always include at least three Complete Breaths and at least a minute or two of meditation.

MAINTENANCE ROUTINE I

After finishing a course, you may wish to practice the techniques for a while before beginning another course. The following routine will keep you in practice until you feel comfortable moving on. It provides essential stretching and strengthening exercises. For variety you can substitute some of the following asans with those that appear in parentheses. Don't forget to incorporate breathing and meditation into your daily practice.

Warm-up Sequence
Easy Balance (Easy Balance Twist)
Tree Pose (Dancer or T Pose)
Standing Rest
Alternate Triangle (Full Triangle)
Standing Sun Pose
Baby Pose
Arm and Leg Balance (Bow Variation)
Cat Breath (Stretching Dog)
Alternate Seated Sun Pose
Spine Twist (Pelvic Twist)
Diamond Pose (Limber Hips)
Cobra Pose
Bow Pose (Boat Pose)
Knee Squeeze
Easy Bridge
Shoulder Stand

COURSE TWO

Introduction

After your first ten weeks of practice, you will have at your disposal a comprehensive repertoire of asans that you can perform smoothly and deliberately. We encourage you to pay attention to details without straining past your capacity.

You should feel comfortable about moving on to the second course if

1. You are practicing at least four days per week.
2. Your complete breath cycle is smooth and correct, using the three stages; the length of each breath is at least 10 seconds in and 10 seconds out (remember, no holding of breath at top or bottom); and each Humming Breath is 3 to 5 seconds in and at least 15 seconds out.
3. You feel comfortable with your relaxation process and practice meditation at least four days per week.
4. You have found a seated position (kneeling, cross-legged, or in a chair) that you can hold comfortably for at least 5 minutes.
5. Your performance of asans is smooth and slow, using the proper breath pattern for each pose.

Please note that there is no standard for limberness. The final position you are able to attain without strain at each point will give you good results.

In this second ten-week course, the objectives are to

1. Limber the hips and knees to improve seated position.
2. Identify breath patterns for each asan.
3. Continue back-strengthening asan work.
4. Learn new breath techniques for stress management, greater quietness, and improved oxygenation.
5. Become familiar with the practice of Asan Point.
6. Build a steady practice schedule of at least 15 minutes per day.
7. Experiment with a seated meditation technique.
8. Learn the Sun Salutation (*Surya Namaskar*) asan sequence.

SHORT ROUTINE FOR BUSY DAYS

For those times when you are feeling energetic but in a pinch for time, this routine will give you essential stretches and strengtheners. It includes more strenuous asans, such as the Cobra and Shoulder Stand, so you must do a full Warm-up Sequence first.

WARM-UP SEQUENCE, p. 24

ALTERNATE TRIANGLE, p. 69

T POSE, p. 78

STANDING SUN POSE, p. 82

BABY POSE, p. 84

ARM AND LEG BALANCE, p. 86

ALTERNATE SEATED SUN POSE, p. 103

PELVIC TWIST, p. 118

COBRA POSE, p. 137

SHOULDER STAND, p. 124

Always include at least three Complete Breaths (p. 150) and at least a minute or two of meditation.

Asan Point

The concept of Asan Point is based on the assumption that asans are 90 percent mental and only 10 percent physical. This means that your attention shifts from the physical pose to a state of mind that is similar to meditation: quiet, focused, and aware. When you have reached a transition point in an asan—for example, the top of the Cobra Pose—stop for a moment (just a second or two). Your body is relaxed, you have checked details such as the correct position of fingers and eyes, your breath is held in or out, and you are not straining. At this point, your mind becomes poised in stillness. Your whole being rests. This is the Asan Point. When you have learned this technique correctly, your entire exercise routine will bring on a state of mind similar to that of meditation.

Breath Patterns in Asans

You may have noticed already that different asans employ different breath patterns. Here are some examples of each.

Complete Breath: Simple in-and-out breaths of even lengths. The Complete Breath pattern allows the greatest volume of air to be inhaled and exhaled. Used with Full Bend, Cobra V-Raise, Arm and Leg Balance, Cat Breath.

Exterior Hold: Short hold at the bottom of the exhalation. This breath pattern is often called a purifying breath. Used with Standing and Seated Sun Poses, Alternate Triangle.

Interior Hold: Short hold at the top of the inhalation. Briefly holding an inhalation allows more oxygen to be absorbed into the bloodstream. Used with Cobra Pose, Bow Pose, Boat Pose.

Interior Compressed Hold: Short hold at the top of the inhalation with compression of midsection. This pattern intensifies the action of the Interior Hold. Used with Easy Balance and Twist, Knee Squeeze.

Easy Breath: A completely nonmanipulated breath pattern, when the breathing muscles are relaxed. In the following examples of very different types of exercises, the rate or intensity of the breath may change, but the breathing muscles are still relaxed. The Easy Breath allows the breath to find its own rhythm as you relax your body in a holding pose. Used with balance poses such as the Dancer Pose, Tree Pose, and T Pose; other holding poses such as the Pigeon Hold, Spine Twist, and Baby Pose.

As an experiment, do your Warm-up Sequence as usual but, instead of going on to your regular asan routine, try each of the asans just listed and focus on how your breathing changes.

WEEKLY CURRICULUM

(*Indicates new exercise*)

WEEK ONE

ASANS

Warm-up Sequence, adding *Hip Rock (p. 67), *Hip Rotation (p. 66), and *Side Triangle (p. 70) after Full Bends

Tree Pose

Dancer Pose

Standing Sun Pose

Arm and Leg Balance

Cat Breath

*Thigh Stretch (p. 96)

Corpse Pose Rest
*Easy Fish Pose (p. 116)
Baby Pose
Back Strengtheners
Knee Squeeze
Easy Bridge
Shoulder Stand
Plow Pose

BREATHING

Breath Warm-ups

Lion

Complete Breath: if length is not up to 10 seconds
in, 10 seconds out, practice breath extension before moving on to the next breath technique

*Kapalabhati (p. 154), 10 seconds bellows; three
complete cycles

MEDITATION

15 to 20 minutes, lying down

WEEK TWO

ASANS

*(As an alternative to the asans listed here, this week
practice identifying breath patterns in the different
asans [see p. 50].)*

Warm-up Sequence
*Twisting Triangle (p. 71)
Tree Pose
Dancer Pose
*T Pose Knee Bends (p. 81)
Standing Sun Pose
*Cobra V-Raise (p. 90)
Baby Pose
Arm and Leg Balance
Cat Breath
Thigh Stretch
Corpse Pose Rest

Easy Fish Pose
Baby Pose
Back Strengtheners
Knee Squeeze
Easy Bridge
Shoulder Stand
Plow Pose

BREATHING

Breath Warm-ups

Lion

*Bramari Breath (p. 156)

Complete Breath, 5 cycles

Kapalabhati, 10 seconds bellows; 3 complete cycles.
Work on evenness of movement and sound.

MEDITATION

15 to 20 minutes. Practice a seated position for
meditation (see p. 144). Concentrate on achieving a fully relaxed body and a stable position.
Hold until you experience discomfort, then finish
lying down.

WEEK THREE

ASANS

Warm-up Sequence
Twisting Triangle
Dancer Pose
Standing Sun Pose
Cobra V-Raise
Alternate Arm and Leg Balance
Cat Breath
Thigh Stretch
Corpse Pose Rest
Fish Pose
*Ankle Stretch (p. 94)
Baby Pose
Knee Squeeze
Easy Bridge

Shoulder Stand
*Sun Salutation (p. 139)

BREATHING

Breath Warm-ups
Lion
*Laughasan (p. 153)
Complete Breath, 5 cycles
Bramari Breath
Kapalabhati, 20 seconds bellows; 3 complete cycles

MEDITATION

15 to 20 minutes, lying down

WEEK FOUR

ASANS

Warm-up Sequence
Tree Pose
Dancer Pose
T Pose Knee Bends
Standing Sun Pose
Arm and Leg Balance
Bow Variation
*Camel Pose (p. 95)
Thigh Stretch
Corpse Pose Rest
*Fish Pose (p. 117)
Ankle Stretch
Baby Pose
*Pigeon Pose and Hold (p. 97)
Back Strengtheners
Knee Squeeze
Easy Bridge
Shoulder Stand
Plow Pose
Sun Salutation

BREATHING

Breath Warm-ups

Lion
Bramari Breath
Kapalabhati, 20 seconds bellows, faster speed; 3 complete cycles

MEDITATION

15 to 20 minutes. Try a seated position for meditation this week; hold until you experience discomfort, then finish lying down.

WEEK FIVE

ASANS

Warm-up Sequence
Tree Pose
Dancer Pose
T Pose Knee Bends
Standing Sun Pose
Arm and Leg Balance
Bow Variation
Camel Pose
Thigh Stretch
Corpse Pose Rest
Fish Pose
Baby Pose
*Hero Pose Variation (p. 92)
*Extended Hero Pose (p. 93)
Pigeon Pose and Hold
Back Strengtheners
Knee Squeeze
*Neck Curl (p. 121)
Easy Bridge
Shoulder Stand
Plow Pose
Sun Salutation

BREATHING

Breath Warm-ups
Lion
Bramari Breath

Kapalabhati, 20 seconds bellows, faster speed; 3
complete cycles

MEDITATION

15 to 20 minutes, lying down

WEEK SIX

ASANS

Warm-up Sequence

Tree Pose

Dancer Pose

T Pose Knee Bends

Standing Sun Pose

Arm and Leg Balance

Cat Breath

Camel Pose

Thigh Stretch

Corpse Pose Rest

Fish Pose

Ankle Stretch

Baby Pose

Hero Pose Variation

Extended Hero Pose

Pigeon Pose and Hold

Back Strengtheners

Knee Squeeze

Neck Curl

*Easy Sit-up (p. 120)

*Sun Pose Balance (p. 102)

Easy Bridge

Shoulder Stand

*Plow Pose Variations (p. 127)

Sun Salutation

BREATHING

*Neti (p. 154)

Breath Warm-ups

Lion

Bramari Breath

Kapalabhati, 20 seconds bellows, faster speed; 3
complete cycles

MEDITATION

15 to 20 minutes. Try seated meditation again this
week.

WEEK SEVEN

ASANS

Warm-up Sequence

*Windmill (p. 72)

Tree Pose

Dancer Pose

T Pose Knee Bends

Standing Sun Pose

Arm and Leg Balance

Cat Breath

Camel Pose

Thigh Stretch

Corpse Pose Rest

Fish Pose

Baby Pose

Spine Twist

Diamond Pose

*Hero Pose (p. 110)

Pigeon Pose and Hold

Back Strengtheners

Knee Squeeze

Neck Curl

Sun Pose Balance

Easy Bridge

Shoulder Stand

Plow Pose

BREATHING

Neti

Breath Warm-ups

Lion

Bramari Breath

Complete Breath, 5 cycles

Kapalabhati, 20 seconds bellows, faster speed; 5
   complete cycles

MEDITATION

15 to 20 minutes. Try seated meditation this week.

WEEK EIGHT

ASANS

   Warm-up Sequence

   Windmill

   Tree Pose

   Dancer Pose

   T Pose Knee Bends

   Standing Sun Pose

   Arm and Leg Balance

   Cat Breath

   Camel Pose

   Thigh Stretch

   Corpse Pose Rest

   Fish Pose

   Baby Pose

   Hero Pose

   Pigeon Pose and Hold

   Back Strengtheners

   Knee Squeeze

   Neck Curl

   *Big Sit-up (p. 122)

   Easy Bridge

   *Alternate Toe Touch (p. 115)

   *The Walk (p. 114)

   Shoulder Stand

   Plow Pose

BREATHING

   Breath Warm-ups

   Lion

Bramari Breath

Kapalabhati, 20 seconds bellows, faster speed; 5
   complete cycles

MEDITATION

   15 to 20 minutes, lying down or seated

WEEK NINE

ASANS

   Warm-up Sequence

   Windmill

   Tree Pose

   Dancer Pose

   T Pose Knee Bends

   Standing Sun Pose

   Alternate Arm and Leg Balance

   Cat Breath

   Camel Pose

   Thigh Stretch

   Corpse Pose Rest

   Fish Pose

   Baby Pose

   Hero Pose

   Pigeon Pose and Hold

   *Airplane Series (p. 133)

   Knee Squeeze

   Neck Curl

   Big Sit-up

   *Easy Bridge with Hold (p. 119)

   Alternate Toe Touch

   The Walk

   Shoulder Stand

   Plow Pose

BREATHING

   Breath Warm-ups

   Lion

   Complete Breath

Bramari Breath

Kapalabhati, 30 seconds bellows, maintain speed; 5
complete cycles

MEDITATION

15 to 20 minutes, seated for at least 5 minutes, the
rest of the time lying down

WEEK TEN

ASANS

Warm-up Sequence

Windmill

Tree Pose

Dancer Pose

T Pose Knee Bends

Standing Sun Pose

Arm and Leg Balance

Cat Breath

Camel Pose

Thigh Stretch

Corpse Pose Rest .

Fish Pose

Baby Pose

Pigeon Pose and Hold

Cobra Pose

Airplane Series

Knee Squeeze

Neck Curl

Big Sit-up

Easy Bridge with Hold

Alternate Toe Touch

Shoulder Stand

Plow Pose

Sun Salutation

BREATHING

Breath Warm-ups

Lion

Complete Breath

Bramari Breath

Kapalabhati, 30 seconds bellows, faster speed; 5
complete cycles

MEDITATION

15 to 20 minutes, seated for at least 5 minutes, the
rest of the time lying down

MAINTENANCE ROUTINE II

Here are two maintenance routines to keep you in
practice after the second course. Alternate them for
best results.

Warm-up Sequence	Warm-up Sequence
Windmill	Windmill
T Pose Knee Bends	Dancer Pose
Standing Sun Pose	Cobra V-Raise
Cobra V-Raise	Thigh Stretch
Baby Pose	Baby Pose
Extended Hero Pose	Sun Salutation
Pigeon Pose and Hold	Corpse Pose Rest
Spine Twist	Knee Squeeze
Seated Sun Pose	Shoulder Stand
Diamond Pose	
Cobra Pose	
Airplane Series	
Neck Curl	
Shoulder Stand	

COURSE THREE

Introduction

If you have been following the curriculum just outlined, you will have been practicing for at least 5 months now. In this third stage of practice you will intensify the format introduced with the Sun Salutation in Course 2. Course 3 emphasizes a routine we call the Emotional Stability Routine.

The objectives of this course are to

1. Learn to recognize the target zones for retention of muscle tension in your body.
2. Strengthen your stomach and back muscles.
3. Increase your stamina.
4. Improve stress resistance.
5. Learn to recognize and release tight breathing patterns.

The Emotional Stability Routine has a direct effect on physical and mental stress reactions. As we will discuss in Chapter 10, we often retain tension or upset after a stressful event because our memory and self-awareness give us the capacity to replay the event again and again in our minds. Every time we replay it, it is etched deeper in our memory.

As we replay that memory, our bodies reexperience their original physiological responses: pulse rate and breathing speed up, blood pressure increases, and hormone messengers are activated. Although our bodies do, more or less, return to a normal state after one of these episodes, our muscles often remain tense and we exhibit other stress responses for extended periods of time—sometimes indefinitely.

This residual tension contributes to stiffness and physical tension. Circulation may be constricted in the head because of tight neck muscles, and we may experience increasing fatigue, lethargy, headaches, and a reduced ability to cope. Emotions become jangled and more out of control as physical constriction leads to mental constriction.

The Emotional Stability Routine counters this syndrome with a group of techniques that act to release physical constriction (and therefore emotional upset and stress responses) in especially vulnerable target areas. With practice this routine can help build resistance to both current and reexperienced stress.

The target zones for the Emotional Stability Routine are (in order of most common tension, pain, or other negative stress response) the stomach, breath muscles, face, upper back and neck, knees, thighs, lower back, throat, and ankles. The Emotional Stability Routine works best when it is practiced every day for the first month, then about two to three times per week. Daily practice in the beginning helps to establish its beneficial effects. You will notice that the Emotional Stability Routine does not include several types of asans—for example, those that work on limberness of hips and knees and those that stretch the fronts of the thighs and the backs of the legs. On the three or four days that you do not practice the Emotional Stability Routine, practice an alternate routine (see example, p. 58) that compensates for these deficits.

An easy version of the Emotional Stability Routine is given at the beginning of this section. Practice it for at least two weeks; then go on to the second version, which adds repetitions and some new exercises. After a minimum of four weeks of practice, you can start the full routine. After six weeks, evaluate the effects of the routine using the Body Talk exercise (p. 44). Talk to different parts of your body, especially the target zones of the Emotional Stability Routine, individually.

WEEKLY CURRICULUM

To maximize its effectiveness, think of the Emotional Stability Routine as more than a series of asans. It is, instead, a sequence of asans, breathing, and meditation.

Emotional Stability Routine, Version I:

WEEKS ONE AND TWO

ASANS

Warm-up Sequence (leave out the Hands and Knees Stretch, since it is included in the main body of asans in this routine)

Windmill (3 each side)

Cobra V-Raise (3)

*Forward Plank (p. 91) (1 each side)

Baby Pose (until breath returns to normal)

*Hands and Knees Stretch with double breath (p. 40) (3)

Cat Breath (3)

Arm and Leg Balance (3 each side)

*Easy Plow Breath (p. 128) (3)

Neck Curl (3)

Alternate Toe Touch (3 each side)

*Side Stretch (p. 111) (1 each side, then reverse feet and repeat)

BREATHING

Complete Breath, 5 cycles

Kapalabhati, 30 seconds bellows; 5 cycles

*Spinal Arch (p. 157) (3)

MEDITATION

Try a seated position for at least 5 minutes, the remainder lying down

Special Note: The Emotional Stability Routine contains strenuous movements that may aggravate a back or neck condition. Do not practice this routine if you have, or suspect you may have, a problem with your spine. If you are not sure, ask your physician for advice. If you start practicing the routine and notice pain in any part of your back, dizziness, headaches, or other unusual symptoms, stop immediately and see your physician.

If you have a back problem and you have your doctor's approval to practice Yoga but are not sure how to proceed without doing the Emotional Stability Routine, please contact us for suggestions (see p. 221).

Emotional Stability Routine, Version II:

WEEKS THREE AND FOUR

ASANS

Warm-up Sequence

Windmill (3 to 6 each side)

Cobra V-Raise (3 to 6)

Forward Plank

*Side Plank (p. 91)

Baby Pose (at least 1 minute, or until breath returns to normal)

Hands and Knees Stretch with double breath

*Cat Breath Variation (p. 88)

Easy Plow Breath (3 to 6)

Walk

Neck Curl

Big Sit-up (instead of, or in addition to, Neck Curl)

Alternate Toe Touch

Side Stretch

BREATHING
  Complete Breath, 5 cycles
  Kapalabhati, 5 cycles
  Spinal Arch
MEDITATION
  At least 5 minutes, seated; total at least 15 minutes

WEEKS FIVE AND SIX

If you have no physical problems with your back, you can begin the full Emotional Stability Routine, alternating with the routine that follows it.

EMOTIONAL STABILITY ROUTINE
  Warm-up Sequence
  Windmill (6 each side)
  Cobra V-Raise (6)
  Forward Plank (1)
  Side Plank (1)
  Baby Pose (1 minute)
  Plow Breath or Easy Plow Breath (6)
  Big Sit-up (6)
  Corpse Pose Rest
  *Alternate Big Sit-up (p. 122) (6 each side)
  Side Stretch (2 each foot position)
  Spinal Arch (3)
ALTERNATE ROUTINE
  Warm-up Sequence
  Twisting Triangle
  Dancer Pose
  T Pose Knee Bends
  Standing Sun Pose or *Sun Pose Variation (p. 85)
  Corpse Pose Rest
  Knee Squeeze
  Alternate Seated Sun Pose
  Limber Hips
  Spine Twist

  Diamond Pose
  Hero Pose
  Extended Hero Pose
  Baby Pose
  Thigh Stretch
  Cat Breath
  Pigeon Pose and Hold
  Cobra Pose
  Shoulder Stand
  Easy Bridge
Breathing
  Kapalabhati, 5 cycles; 45 seconds bellows
  *Agni Kriya (p. 158)
Meditation
  At least 10 minutes, seated

WEEK SEVEN

Earlier we talked about how the Emotional Stability Routine is meant to affect the body's target zones that respond to stress by holding or tightening the respiratory and other muscles. This week, at least once, go back to the Body Talk exercise (see p. 44) and have a written dialogue with your body. Decide which areas of your body you wish to communicate with and focus on them. Then talk to your body as a whole concerning the physical and emotional effects the routine has brought about.

Begin by talking to your breath. What physical changes have occurred since you began practicing this routine? Have you noticed any changes in the way your breath responds to stress? Now talk to your stomach. How does it feel? Are its muscles any stronger than before? Does it feel more resilient to tension? Does it get upset as often? Now talk to your face. How has your face responded to the physical and emotional effects of this routine? When you look in the mirror, does your face look different? How? Does it feel more in control of its muscular reactions? Does it feel any more relaxed? Move on to your neck and throat. Does your throat constrict when tense? Any less so since beginning this routine? Are you feeling better able to express your thoughts and feelings? Now move to your lower back. Does it feel stronger? Does it feel any more limber? If you have had chronic pain or stiffness in your back, has that improved at all? Does your lower back feel more comfortable when you sit for meditation? Move along to your hips and thighs. Are they feeling stronger? More limber? Do you feel freer when you walk or run? If you have been bothered with cramping in your legs, has that improved? Talk to your knees. Do they feel stronger? Better able to support you? Are they free from mysterious aches and pains? Do they complain as much when you are in a seated position for meditation or breathing? Finally, talk to your ankles. Do they feel stronger and more supportive? Do they bother you when you sit cross-legged?

Talk to your body as a whole. How does it adapt to stressful conditions? Has it learned better responses than before? Does it recover faster? Do you sleep better? Is your metabolism functioning normally? Do you have enough energy to do what you want to do? How is your posture? Does your body have any complaints about the food you are feeding it? About the kinds of activities you do in addition to Yoga? About Yoga practice? What does your body like most about the Emotional Stability Routine? Least? How can you and your body work together to get the most out of this routine? Continue alternating between the two routines outlined for Weeks 5 and 6.

WEEK EIGHT

This week experiment doing the routines at different speeds. Asan sequences in Yoga can be practiced quickly, with shorter, more intense breathing patterns, or more slowly, with longer breath cycles and brief holds at each Asan Point. The faster version of the Emotional Stability Routine, which takes 7 to 10 minutes, demands that your body change its breathing pattern rapidly; thus your mood can be shifted more easily. The slower version (which takes about 20 minutes) reinforces a concentrated state of mind; your attention is focused on the transition points.

When you are practicing the routine at the faster speed, pay careful attention to the details, such as the position of hands and feet, and breathe as much air in and out as before. The idea is to move and breathe a little faster, but not carelessly. In the slower version, take care not to hold your breath so long at the transition points that you gasp for air. Remember that the full routine includes breathing and meditation as well as the asans.

WEEK NINE

This week vary your alternate routine to include asans that you have not practiced in a while. Include the Sun Salutation especially, and practice this routine in both faster and slower versions if you can. Experiment with creating several other alternate routines for yourself. Your goal is to achieve a balance of stretches and strengtheners.

WEEK TEN

This week do the Body Talk exercise again, asking the same questions of the different parts of your body (and any new questions that occur to you). See if there has been any change from the last time you did the exercise.

Experiment with the following routine in order to practice holding Yoga asans for an extended period. Do not practice this routine more than two days in a row. When the routine instructs you to hold a position in which you usually hold the breath in or out, change to a relaxed breath for the holding period. As you come out of the hold, return to the normal breath pattern to finish the exercise. For example, if you are holding the Seated Sun Pose at the bottom, when your breath is normally held out, release the breath and just relax into the pose. You may have to grasp your legs a bit higher to avoid strain during the hold. When you are ready to come out of the hold, breathe in to a count of three as you raise your arms up in a circle overhead, then breathe out to a count of three as you lower your arms to your sides. When holding, adjust the position of your head, if necessary, to prevent strain to your neck.

Do not strain. If the suggested holding intervals cause shakiness, fatigue, or muscle pain, reduce the length of each hold. Balance poses often reveal strain; a shaking body indicates that your nervous system has had enough. The length of time that you can hold a position will vary from day to day, depending on your stress levels, fatigue, nutrition, moods, and other factors, so do not be discouraged if you cannot hold a position as long as you did the day before. Each day's effort—even if it seems less than the previous day's—will contribute to steady improvements in your strength and balance. Remember that the idea is to achieve a relaxed stretch, keeping the breath pattern smooth and relaxed and the mind poised and still.

ROUTINE FOR PRACTICING HOLDING POSITIONS

Warm-up Sequence—Regular speed.

Alternate Triangle—Hold each leg at the bottom stretch for 15 seconds. Switch to relaxed breath while holding.

Standing Rest—Hold 30 to 60 seconds.

Dancer Pose—Hold each side for 30 seconds. Be sure to relax the stomach muscles. Switch to relaxed breath while holding.

Standing Sun Pose—Regular speed.

Baby Pose—Hold 30 to 60 seconds.

Cobra V-Raise—Hold each transition (extreme up and extreme down) for 3 seconds. (Do not relax breath in these short holds.)

Baby Pose—Hold 30 to 60 seconds.

Pigeon Pose and Hold—Hold 30 seconds. Switch to relaxed breath while holding.

Cat Breath—Hold each extreme position for 3 seconds. (Do not relax breath in these short holds.)

Arm and Leg Balance—Hold alternate arm and leg up for 10 seconds. Switch to relaxed breath while holding.

Easy Cobra Pose—Regular speed.

Alternate Seated Sun Pose—Hold downward position for 15 seconds. Switch to relaxed breath while holding.

Shoulder Stand—Hold 30 to 60 seconds.

AFTER COURSE THREE . . .

If you have been following the courses outlined in this chapter, you have now been practicing Yoga for more than seven months. You have learned more than seventy asans, several breathing techniques, and a procedure for relaxation and meditation. How do you choose which techniques to practice each day?

You have already learned several routines: the Maintenance Routines and the Emotional Stability Routine, among others. You may choose from any of these—or from any of the weekly routines for any course—to add variety to your daily practice. You may also create your own routines. Be sure always to include some exercise, some breathing, and some meditation for a well-balanced daily practice.

If you have questions about your personal curriculum, please contact us (see p. 221), and we will try our best to help you continue your Yoga practice most productively.

Chapter 4

EXERCISE (ASANA)

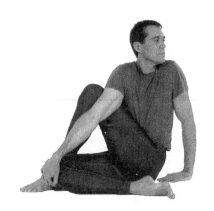

This chapter illustrates and describes each asan listed in the course curricula of Chapter 3 and lists the benefits of each. Before you attempt any asans, be sure you have warmed up by following the sequence in Chapter 2. The asans are organized from standing to kneeling to sitting to prone. More advanced asans and variations are placed alongside the easier versions. Each asan is labeled Course 1, 2, and/or 3, referring to the course curriculum in which the asan appears. Some asans are repeated in more than one course.

Remember to read through each exercise before you try it. If you have a physical limitation, you may need to modify the exercise in order to perform it comfortably. Remember to move slowly and deliberately, and do not strain. The benefit of practicing Yoga asans derives not only from moving the body in a prescribed way but also from coordinating the physical movement with the breath pattern and aiming for a concentrated mind.

As you follow the course curricula in Chapter 3, go at your own pace. The weekly routines are suggestions only. If you are elderly or have physical limitations, proceed even more slowly than usual to give your body time to get used to the movements. You may have to simplify the positions somewhat. Be creative. Yoga is not a rigid process but a fluid one, allowing every individual to find his or her own pace and intensity.

Rest Poses
- Relax entire body

After every three or four asans, rest for 30 to 60 seconds to one minute to allow your muscles to relax and your breath to return to normal. Close your eyes and quickly check your body's most troublesome tension spots: eyes, jaw, stomach, and so on. Let yourself go completely limp. If it helps, imagine that you are a rag doll.

STANDING REST

Stand with your feet parallel (A); separate them a few inches if it helps you balance. Relax your arms at your sides. Close your eyes and try to balance equally on both feet. Keep your spine straight; imagine that there is a string attached to the top of your head, pulling you upright. Pay extra attention to your facial muscles, your shoulders, and your stomach, trying to relax as much as possible.

CORPSE POSE REST (SHAVASAN)

Lie down on your mat, arms at your sides or slightly out from your body, with palms facing up (B). With eyes closed, relax your face, your shoulders, your stomach, and any other areas of your body that hold tension.

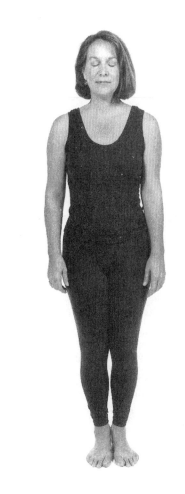

A

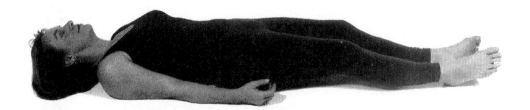

B

Easy Balance (Course I)

- Improves circulation and respiration
- Strengthens nervous system
- Improves balance and concentration
- Strengthens leg muscles, including calves and ankles
- Helps relieve sciatica and leg cramps

Stand with arms at your sides (A). Now breathe in to a count of three as you bring your arms out slightly and rise on your toes. Make fists and press them into your diaphragm—just below the rib cage (B). Fix your gaze on one spot to help you balance, and hold your breath for a count of three. Then breathe out to a count of three as you come back down on your heels, arms relaxed at your sides. Concentrate on fluidity of movement as you do repetitions. Repetitions: 3 to 5.

Stare at one spot for balance.
Make fists just under your rib cage.
Lift and lower your heels slowly.

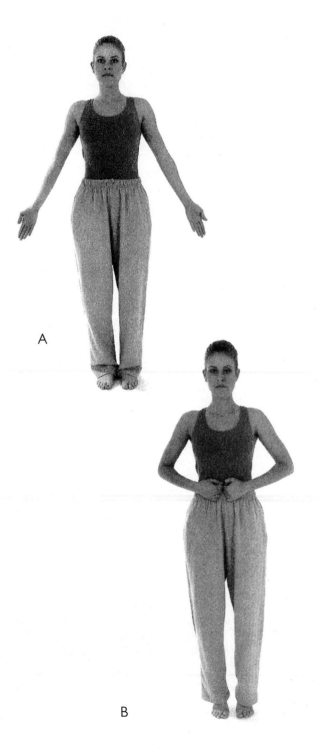

A

B

Easy Balance Twist (Course 1)

- Improves circulation
- Expands chest and lungs
- Develops steadiness and poise
- Strengthens calves, ankles, and toes

Stand with arms at your sides. Breathe in to a count of three as you rise on your toes, bringing your arms in a wide circle to the sides and overhead. Press your palms together (A). Steady yourself by fixing your gaze on one spot. Hold your breath in to a count of three as you twist to the right, finding another spot to fix your gaze on (B). Twist with your whole body, not just your torso. Then breathe out as you count to three and turn back to the front, bring your arms back down to the sides in a circle, lower your heels to the floor, and relax. Repeat on the left side. Repetitions: 3 to each side, alternating.

If you find it difficult to keep your balance as you twist, lower your heels and rest a moment before you lift again and continue. Do this as many times as needed wherever you are in the exercise sequence.

Breathe fully and deeply through your nose.
Stare at one spot for balance.
Press your palms together overhead.
Twist your whole body, not just your torso.

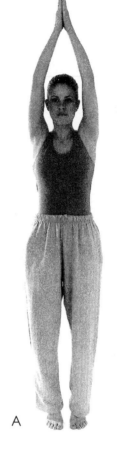

A

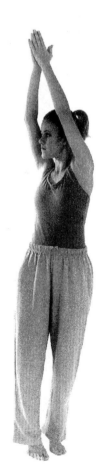

B

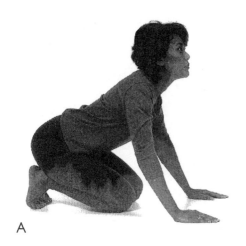

A

Stretching Dog (Course 1)
(Adho Mukhasvanasan)

- Limbers shoulder joints, hip joints, and tendons in lower legs
- Helps reduce arthritic pain and stiffness in shoulders
- Relieves fatigue
- Stretches backs of legs and spine
- Increases circulation to head and eyes
- Improves overall circulation

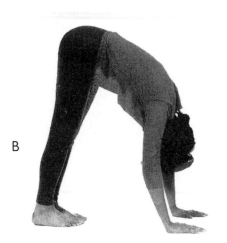

B

Sit on your heels with toes tucked under and hands on the floor a few inches in front of your knees. Breathe in to a count of three as you look up, creating a very slight arch in your back (A). Hold for a count of three. Now breathe out to a count of three as you push up into a V, straightening your legs as much as possible and pushing your heels toward the floor (B). Be careful not to strain. Tuck your head under. Now breathe in and lower back into the start position. Repetitions: 3 to 5.

Breathe deeply through your nose.
Tuck your head under.
Slowly try to straighten your legs without strain.

Hip Rotation (Courses 2 & 3)

- Limbers hip joints, lower back, and upper thighs

In Courses 2 and 3 add this to the Warm-up Sequence after the Full Bend. Separate your feet a comfortable distance, but keep your toes pointed forward or slightly inward at all times. Place your hands on your hips, thumbs hooked forward over your hipbones and fingers spread over the lower back for support (A, next page). (This support will help prevent possible injury from bending backward too far.)

Slowly rotate your hips 360 degrees several times in each direction. Try to stretch the upper thighs and hips as much as possible without strain.

Keep torso straight.
Keep your feet parallel, toes pointed straight forward or slightly inward.
Breathe normally.
Support your lower back.

Hip Rock (Courses 2 & 3)

- Limbers hip joints and lower back
- Stretches backs of legs
- Strengthens lower back
- Massages digestive organs
- Relieves tension in back and neck

In Courses 2 and 3, add this exercise to the Warm-up Sequence after the Hip Rotation. Starting in the same position as Hip Rotation (A), breathe in to a count of three as you push your hips forward slightly (B), keeping your head straight (do not drop it back), then breathe out to a count of three as you bend forward, letting your arms drop to the floor or as far forward as possible (C). Relax your head, neck, arms, and back completely and hold your breath out for a count of three. Now breathe in to a count of three as you come back up, replacing your hands on your hips and pushing forward. Repeat this pumping motion in coordination with the breath. Repetitions: 3 to 5.

Move slowly and deliberately.
Breathe fully, through nose.
Support your lower back.

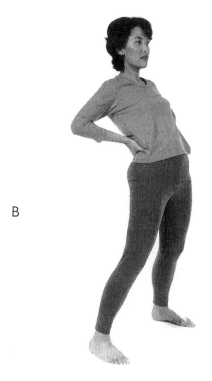

B

Keep your toes pointed forward or slightly inward.

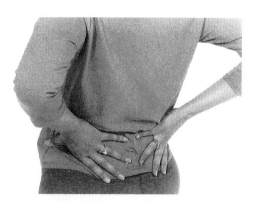

A

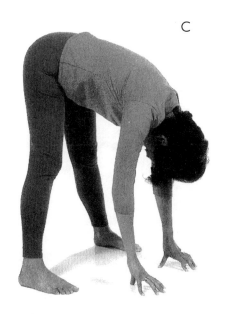

C

Full Triangle (Course 1)
(Prasarita Padottanasan)

- Limbers and strengthens hamstrings and abductor muscles
- Improves circulation and functioning of the kidneys, spleen, stomach, intestines, heart, and lungs
- Improves circulation

Standing with your feet apart, toes pointed in, breathe in to a count of three as you open your arms to the sides (A). Breathe out to a count of three as you bend forward, hands toward the floor (B). Grasp both ankles or calves and pull gently (C). Hold for a count of three, then release, cross your arms, and hang gently, breathing normally, for a few seconds; eventually you will become so limber that you can rest your crossed arms on the floor (D). Repetitions: 1.

Keep your toes pointed in.

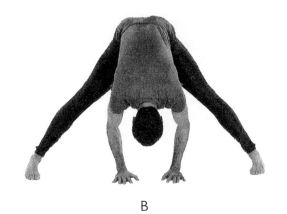

B

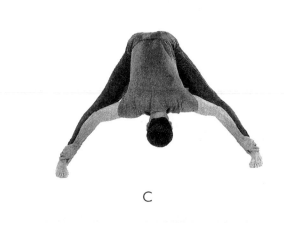

C

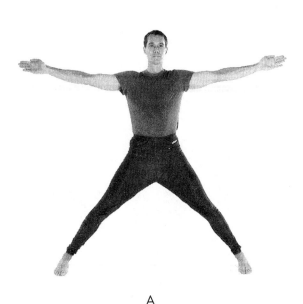

A

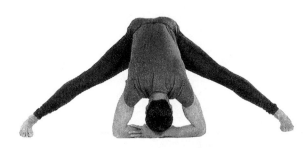

D

Alternate Triangle (Course 1)
(Trikona Hasthasan)

- Localizes and stretches ligaments and nerves in legs, back, shoulders, and neck
- Improves circulation in the entire pelvic region
- Reduces body fat
- Massages internal organs
- Improves circulation to face and eyes

Separate your feet a comfortable distance, with toes pointed forward or slightly inward. To warm up, bend forward gently, first to the center, then to each leg, to be sure that you will not be straining your back. Slowly straighten up.

Breathe in to a count of three as you stretch your arms wide, parallel to the floor (A). Now breathe out to a count of three as you slowly bend down to your right leg (E). Grasp the leg with both hands, bend your elbows, keeping your arms close to your body, and gently pull your upper body toward your leg. Hold your breath out for a count of three. (If you can't bend your elbows, grasp your leg a little higher up. The idea is to pull the upper body by using the arms rather than by using the stomach or lower back muscles, which might cause strain.) Then breathe in to a count of three as you slowly return to a standing position with arms outstretched. Repetitions: 3 to each side, alternating.

Breathe deeply and completely.
Grip your legs firmly as you pull.
Move slowly—take 4 to 5 seconds for each
    movement.

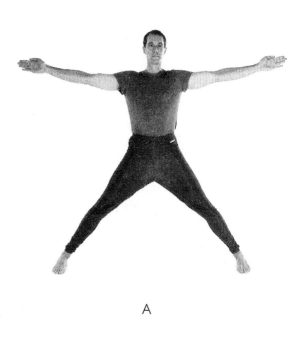

A

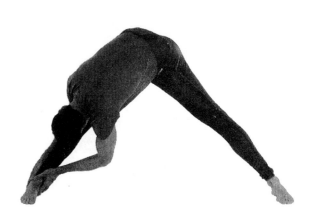

E

Side Triangle (Courses 2 & 3)
(Uttihita Trikonasan)

- Tones muscles of legs and hips
- Stretches respiratory muscles
- Helps relieve backaches
- Strengthens neck

In Courses 2 and 3 add this exercise to the Warm-up Sequence after the Hip Rock. Stand with your feet apart a comfortable distance, toes pointed slightly in. Lift your arms straight out to the sides (A). Breathe in to a count of three as you bend to the right, sliding your right hand down your leg as far as possible without strain (F). Grip your leg for support. At the same time bring your left arm up and over your head so it is as parallel as possible to the floor and in a plane with the rest of your body. Hold your breath in for a count of three, then breathe out to a count of three as you straighten up to the start position (A), with your arms straight out to the sides. Repeat on the left side. Repetitions: 3 on each side, alternating.

After you have been practicing this exercise for at least four months, you may start holding the position a little longer. At this point do not hold your breath in, but relax and breathe easily in the position.

Keep your toes pointed in slightly.
Have your upper arm as straight as possible, parallel to the floor, and in a plane with the rest of your body.

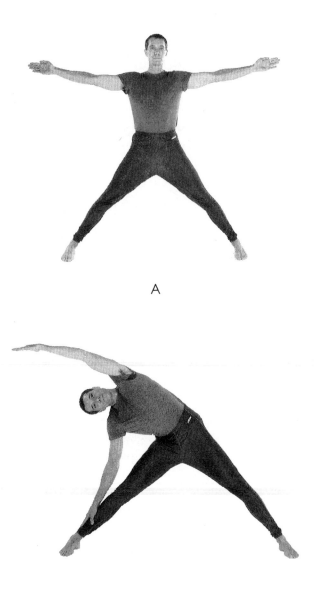

A

F

Twisting Triangle (Courses 2 & 3)
(Parivritta Trikonasan)

- Increases flexibility and blood circulation in lower spine and pelvis
- Strengthens hip joints
- Massages internal organs
- Strengthens chest and neck
- Helps relieve depression

With your legs apart 2 to 3 feet or a comfortable distance and your toes pointed in, breathe in to a count of three as you raise your arms straight out to the sides (A). Breathe out to a count of three as you bend forward from the hips and toward your right leg. Tilt your pelvis forward rather than leading with your head. As you bend, twist your torso clockwise. Grasp the outside of your right calf, ankle, or foot with your left hand and pull slightly as you twist even more, raising your right arm straight up (G). Keep your eyes open and look up at your right thumbnail. Hold for a count of three, then return to a standing position, breathing in to a count of three as you come up. Move slowly and deliberately. Repeat on the left side.

> Grasp the outside of your calf, ankle, or foot with the opposite hand.
> Breathe out as you twist downward, in as you come up.
> Look at your upraised thumbnail.

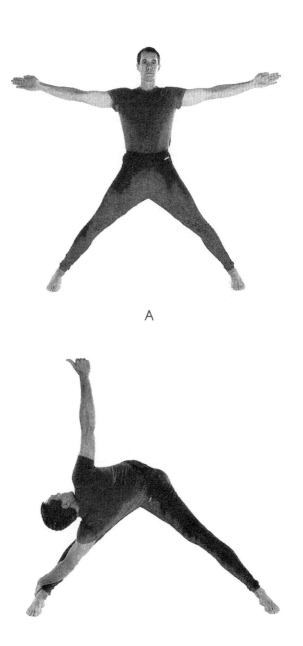

A

G

Windmill (Courses 2 & 3)

- Limbers and strengthens lower spine, hip joints, and muscles of upper thighs
- Improves respiration

Start with your feet apart, toes pointed in, hands supporting your lower back with fingers spread (A). Breathe in to a count of three as you swivel to the right without moving your feet, so that your torso is facing right (B). Breathe out to a count of three as you bend forward toward your right leg (C). Bend as far down toward the leg as possible but don't stop; continue moving down and over to your left leg, still breathing out (D). At this point your breath should be all the way out. When your head reaches the position of your left leg, start breathing in to a count of three as you straighten up, eventually facing left (E). When you reach a standing position, your breath should be all the way in and you will be facing left. Hold the breath in to a count of three as you swivel right and repeat the exercise. Repetitions: 3 in each direction.

Notice that in this exercise your head describes a circle. You breathe out for two-thirds of the circle (from straight up to the left leg) and you breathe in for one-third of the circle (left leg up to straight position). If this breath pattern seems familiar, it should. It's the Humming Breath—short inhalation, long exhalation (p. 152).

Breathe in and out completely.
Swivel completely to each side before and after making the circle.
Keep your knees straight.
Support your lower back with spread fingers.

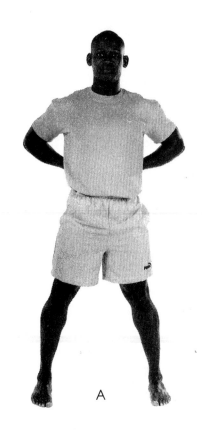

A

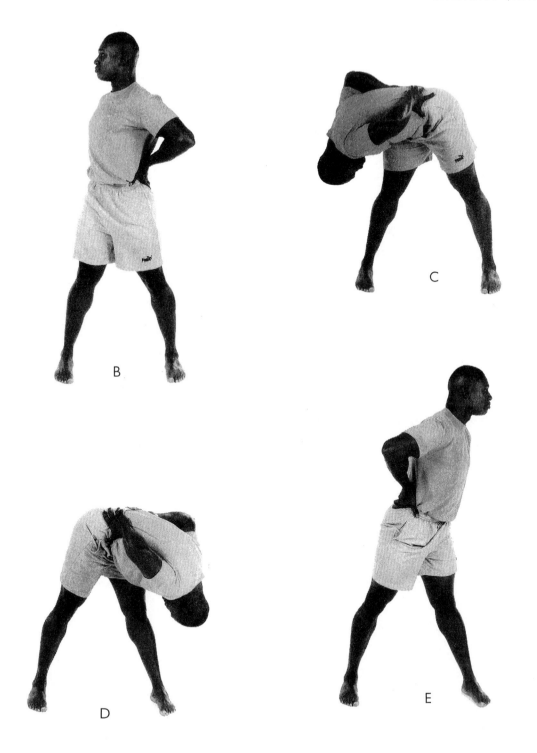

B

C

D

E

Tree Pose (Courses 1 & 2)
(Vriksasan)

- Strengthens legs
- Enhances concentration and balance
- Improves respiration

Stand with your feet together. To get the feeling of balancing on one leg, first shift your weight to your left foot and rest your right foot on top of the left. Steady yourself by fixing your gaze on a spot on the wall or floor in front of you. At first hold on to the back of a chair, a bar, or the wall—something solid. Now pick up your right foot and place it against the inside of your left leg as high as possible, with the toes pointed toward the floor (A). You may find it easier to hold your foot in place if you are barefoot. If your foot will not go high enough to rest on your inner thigh, just brace it against your knee.

Try to breathe steadily, with relaxed stomach muscles, for the duration of the pose. Because of the extra concentration required to maintain your balance, you may find that you tend to hold your breath. Consciously relax your breath by relaxing your stomach muscles.

When you feel that your balance is steady enough to let go of your support, slowly bring your arms straight up overhead with palms together (B). Keep breathing normally. Hold for about 10 seconds at first; work up to 30 seconds or more. Repetitions: 1 each side.

Eventually, as your flexibility increases, your lifted leg will become more parallel to the rest of your body. In the beginning it's more important to concentrate on maintaining a balanced pose than to worry about the position of the lifted leg. On unsteady days, try placing one upraised arm against a wall or doorframe to steady yourself.

Variation: After you have been practicing for some time, your hips and knees will begin to limber up, and you may be able to place your foot on top of your opposite thigh (C). If so, keep your supporting leg straight and slightly tilt your pelvis forward. As your limberness improves, you will be able to lower your knee toward your supporting leg. Your arms are straight overhead, palms together, as before. This variation strengthens the knee joints.

Variation: If you feel very steady, you can try a variation in which you look up slightly as you balance. Be sure to keep your stomach muscles relaxed so that your breath can relax.

Stare at one spot.
Relax your stomach muscles for relaxed breathing.
Keep your arms straight overhead.

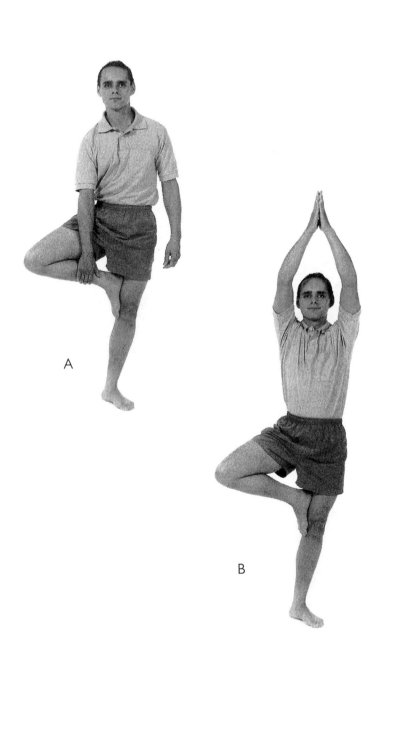

A

B

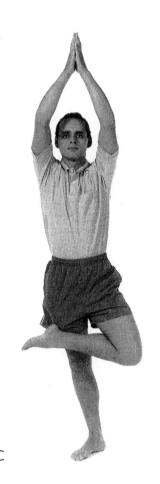

C

Dancer Pose (Courses 1, 2, & 3)
(Natarajasan)

- Strengthens lower back and lumbar vertebrae
- Stretches and strengthens hips and thighs
- Improves balance, poise, and concentration
- Removes phlegm and opens nasal passages
- Improves memory
- Helps relieve sluggishness and depression

If you have lower back or neck problems, check with your doctor before attempting this exercise.

Fix your eyes on one spot for balance. Grasp your right foot firmly with your left hand (A). Raise your right arm straight overhead, pointed toward the ceiling, next to your ear (B). Now lift your right leg up and back away from your body (not just in toward the buttocks) slowly and carefully (C). Re-

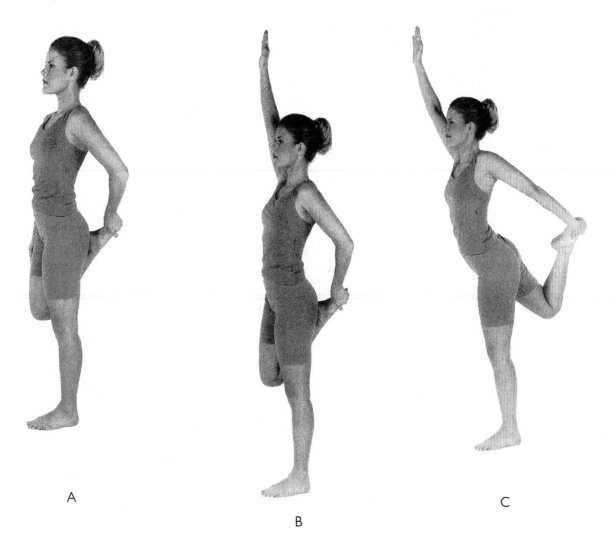

A

B

C

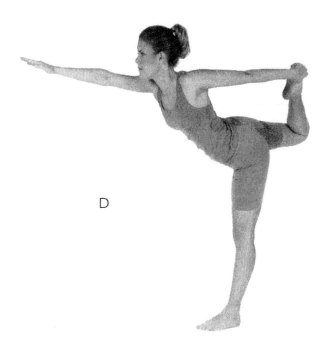

D

lax your stomach muscles so that you feel your breath mostly in the diaphragm. Hold the position, relaxing your stomach muscles and breathing easily, for several seconds. When you feel steady, slowly bend forward, keeping your upraised leg pulled away from your body as much as possible and looking forward at your out-stretched hand (D). Then relax and repeat once on the left side. If your balance is shaky, hold on to a doorframe or lean against a wall (E).

Stare at one spot for balance.

Grasp your opposite foot.

Release your stomach muscles so that the breath re-laxes.

Pull your foot up and push it back away from the body.

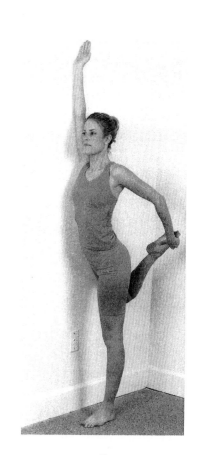

E

T Pose (Courses 1, 2, & 3)
(Virabhadrasan)

- Develops strong legs, back, and nervous system
- Enhances vigor and agility and may improve eyesight
- Reduces anxiety
- Massages internal organs and may improve kidney function
- Increases concentration and mental poise

Holding on to a sturdy chair, step back from the chair about 3 feet. Lower your torso so that it is parallel to the floor. Raise and lower each leg a few times to warm up and get a feeling for holding your leg straight out to the back (A).

Raise your right leg and bring it as high as you can without bending either of your knees. Now fix your gaze on a spot on the floor, relax your stomach muscles and find your center of balance by gradually releasing your hold on the chair. Bring your palms together with fingers pointed straight down toward the floor (B). Hold for a few seconds, then relax and repeat on the left side. Keep your neck straight.

You may also start this exercise by resting both hands on your supporting knee. Stare at a spot on the floor and slowly raise your right leg behind you until it is parallel to the floor or as high as you can lift it without straining (C). Keep both knees straight. Then, when you feel steady, bring your hands together as described before.

After you have practiced this exercise for a few weeks, you can go on to the completed pose, with arms straight out in front, palms together (D). Gaze at your outstretched hands. In this position your arms, torso, raised leg, and supporting leg should all be straight.

Relax your stomach muscles.
Keep your legs, torso, and arms straight.

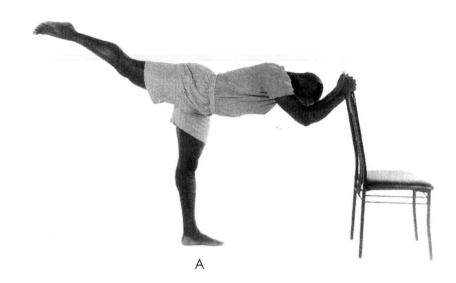

A

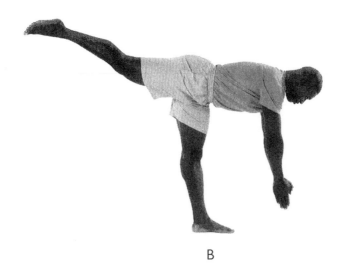

B

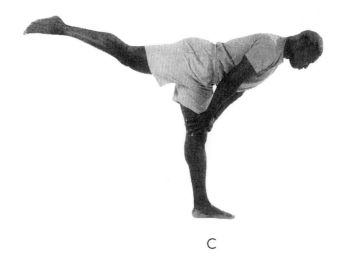

C

T Pose Variations
(*Virabhadrasan* Variation)

After practicing these balance poses for some time, you may wish to go on to some more advanced stretches. In one variation, from position (D) you'll bend your arms, keeping your palms together, get your balance, and turn your torso and raised leg to the side, attempting to bring your arms into the plane of your body (E).

In another variation, the Stork Stretch (*Urdhva Prasarita Ekapadasan*), after holding the T Pose, drop your arms so that your fingers or palms touch the ground. Your lifted leg stays parallel to the floor or higher (F).

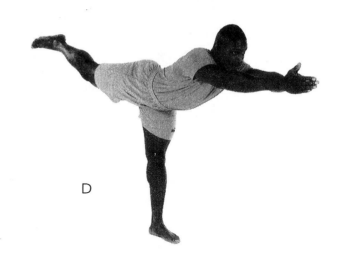

D

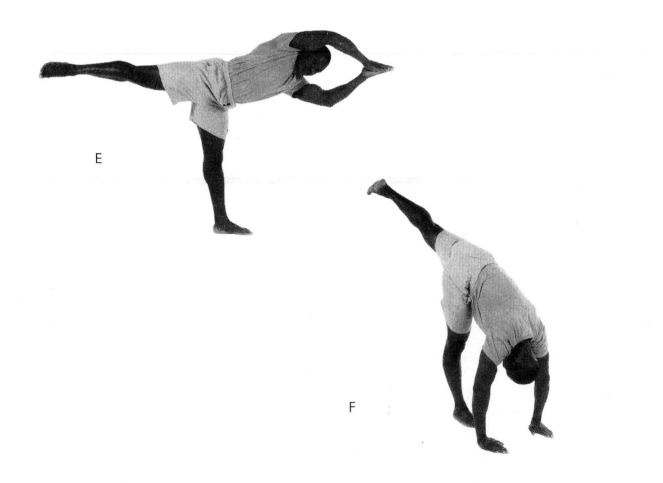

E

F

T Pose Knee Bends
(Courses 2 & 3)

- Strengthen hips, knees, lower back, and legs
- Improve concentration, steadiness, and balance

From the T Pose, bring your arms behind your back and clasp your hands (G). Rest them comfortably on your buttocks. Now stare at one spot for balance and gently bend the knee of your supporting leg. Bend only a few inches—this is not meant to be a deep knee bend. Repeat on the opposite side. Repeat, trying for 5 repetitions at first. After several weeks you may increase to 10. If your balance is unsteady, use a chair for support (H).

Keep your hands loosely clasped.
Keep your breathing relaxed.

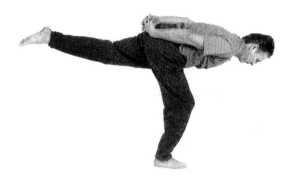

G

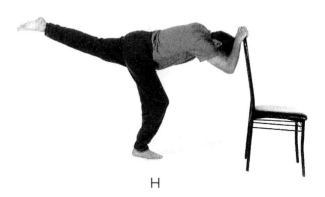

H

Standing Sun Pose (Courses 1, 2, & 3) (Padahasthasan)

- Stimulates stomach, liver, spleen, and other internal organs
- Improves circulation
- Strengthens respiration
- Limbers and strengthens muscles and nerves in back and legs

Stand straight, feet parallel, and breathe out to a count of three (A). Breathe in to a count of three as you raise your arms to the sides in a circle (B) and then overhead with palms together. Stretch and look up (C). Hold for a count of three. Then breathe out to a count of three as you bend forward from the hips, keeping your head between your outstretched arms (D). Try to match your breath to your movement so that your breath is not all the way out until you are all the way down. Hold your breath out for a count of three as you grasp your calves firmly with both hands; bend your elbows, keeping your arms close to your sides, and pull your upper body gently toward your legs (E). Pull with your arms, not your stomach or back muscles. If

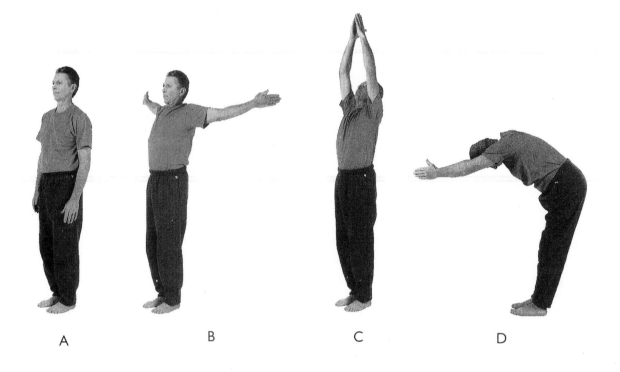

A   B   C   D

you can't bend your elbows, grasp your legs farther up until you can bend them. Now release your legs and breathe in to a count of three as you straighten up, keeping your arms loose at first, then out to the sides (F) and overhead again, so that your breath is all the way in when your arms are overhead. Then breathe out to a count of three as you lower your arms to your sides. Relax. Repetitions: 3.

When you are more limber, you may be able to pull your upper body even farther toward your legs (G). In the completed pose, the face, not the top of the head, touches the legs.

Unlike the other forward-bending poses learned so far, this exercise does not have a continuous up-and-down motion. Instead you must lower your arms between each repetition.

Keep your knees straight.
Pull by bending the elbows, not by tensing the stomach or back.
Coordinate movement with breath.
Bend slowly.

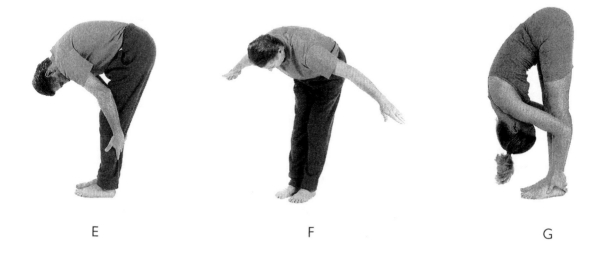

E   F   G

Baby Pose

- Limbers lower back
- Reduces body fat from sides and hips
- Improves circulation in pelvic region
- Improves digestion
- Strengthens knees and ankles
- Relieves stiffness in hips, knees, and ankles
- Enhances functioning of reproductive system

Do not do this exercise if you have high blood pressure.

Sit on your heels with your toes flat against the floor (A). Bend forward until your head touches the floor. If that is comfortable, bend your arms back, elbows out to the sides, so that your neck and shoulders can relax (B). Your elbows should be resting on the floor. Your head can rest on the floor on your forehead, the bridge of your nose, or the crown—whatever is comfortable. However, your neck should be straight; avoid turning your head to one side. Breathe normally and relax as much as possible. Wiggle around and find the most comfortable position.

If putting your head on the floor creates too much abdominal discomfort, try these variations: (1) separate your knees several inches to a foot; (2) cross your arms in front of your knees and rest your head on your arms (C); (3) rest your crossed arms on your knees and bend your head forward, being sure to relax the back of the neck.

If your hips or knees are too stiff for this position, try a variation of this exercise called the Folded Pose, using a chair (see p. 203). Sit with your hips against the back of the chair, feet flat, knees slightly apart. Bend forward and let your arms relax over your ankles. (Your arms may also be crossed on your knees if you experience discomfort from ab-

dominal compression.) Be sure to relax your neck completely.

Relax completely.

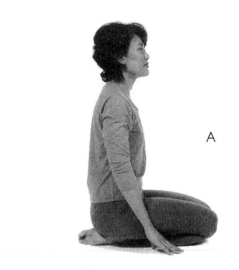

A

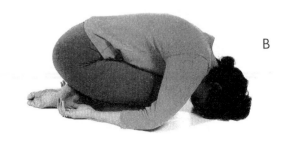

B

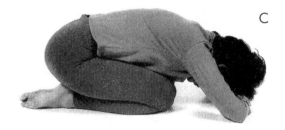

C

Sun Pose Variation (Course 3)
(Parsvottanasan)

- Limbers shoulder joints and shoulder blades, lumbar vertebrae, and neck
- Gives intense stretch to respiratory muscles
- Helps correct breathing difficulties
- Massages internal organs
- Strengthens legs and back
- Improves posture

This variation of the Standing Sun Pose is for those who are rather limber and can attempt a more challenging pose. Your hands are clasped behind your back, arms straight and flexed up and away from the body. This position is common to several other advanced Yoga asans. It limbers all the upper back muscles and joints, as well as stretching the rib cage and lungs, allowing more freshly oxygenated blood into the nerves and tissues of the heart and lungs.

Stand straight, with hands clasped and arms locked behind your back (A). Breathe in deeply to a count of three, then breathe out to a count of three as you bend forward from the hips. Flex your arms up and away from your back. Bend forward as far as possible, bringing your upper body close to your legs without bending your knees (B). Hold this position with the breath out for a count of three, then breathe in to a count of three as you come up. Repetitions: 3.

Clasp your hands and lock your elbows.
Bend slowly and breathe deeply.
Keep your knees straight.

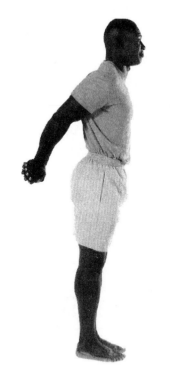

A

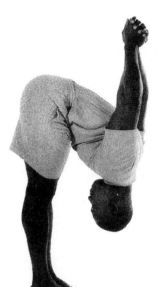

B

Arm and Leg Balance (Courses 1, 2, & 3)

- Strengthens hip joints
- Improves balance
- Promotes correct posture
- Strengthens shoulders and upper back

Starting on your hands and knees, breathe in to a count of three as you slowly raise your left arm and right leg (A). Try to lift the arm straight out in front of you and the leg straight out in back, so both are parallel to the floor. Hold for a count of three, looking at the tip of your middle finger, then breathe out to a count of three as you lower your arm and leg. If your balance is a bit shaky at first, focus on a spot on the floor. Repeat with the opposite arm and leg. Repetitions: 3 on each side, alternating sides.

Variation: Raise the left arm and left leg (B). Try not to lean to the side; keep the back as straight and level as possible. Repeat on the right side. Repetitions: 3 on each side, alternating sides.

Gaze at a spot on the floor for balance, or at the tip of your outstretched middle finger.

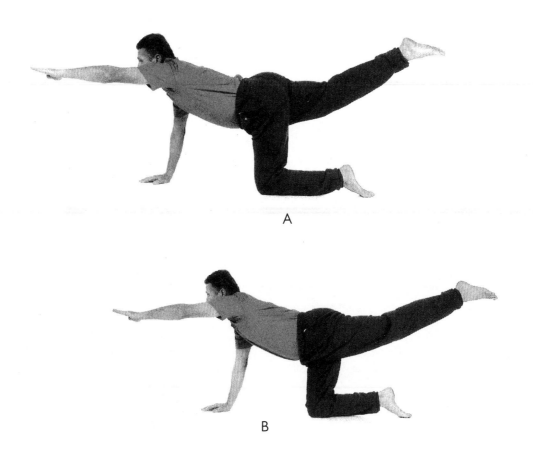

A

B

Cat Breath (Courses 1, 2, & 3)

- Improves digestion and circulation
- Helps manage hypertension
- Limbers spinal column and relieves tension in lower back
- Improves respiration and strengthens breathing muscles

Start on your hands and knees (A). Breathe in to a count of three as you arch your back and look up (B). Then breathe out to a count of three as you tuck your head, rounding your back so your spine bends in the opposite direction (C). Repetitions: 3 to 5.

Breathe deeply and smoothly.
Coordinate the breath with the movement of your spine.

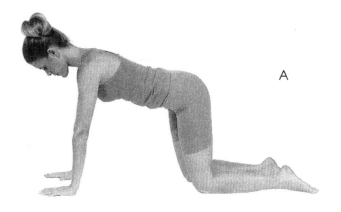

A

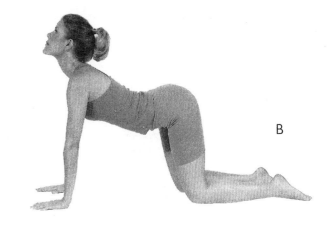

B

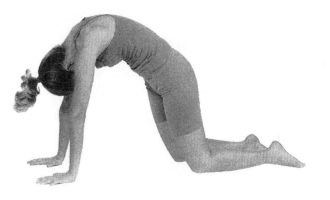

C

Cat Breath Variation (Course 3)

- Breaks up tense breathing patterns
- Strengthens upper back, shoulders, and hip joints
- Limbers lower spine

This exercise is part of the Emotional Stability Routine (Course 3). It involves using a "double breath," meaning that the breath is manipulated by the natural movement of the body. Start on your hands and knees and breathe in to a count of three (A). Breathe out to a count of three as you tuck your head under and bring your left knee up toward your forehead (B). This is a natural breath; bringing your forehead and knee together compresses your midsection, forcing air from your lungs. Now breathe in to a count of three as you raise your head and extend your leg back (C). Continue lifting your leg as high as possible, while breathing out to a count of three and simultaneously bending your elbows and arching your back so that your chin comes toward the floor (D). This movement also naturally expels air from your lungs. As you gain proficiency in this breath pattern, you can speed up the movement. Repeat with your right knee. Repetitions: 3 to 6 with each leg.

Breathe out in the extreme up and extreme down positions, and breathe in during the transitions.

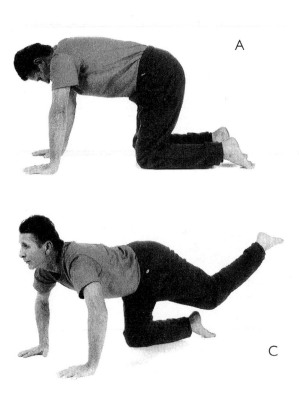

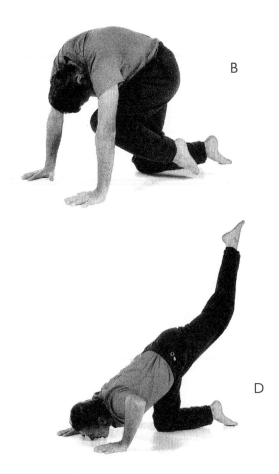

Bow Variation (Courses 1 & 2)
(*Dhanurasan* Variation)

- Strengthens spine, back muscles, hips, thighs, and shoulders
- Improves balance and memory

Starting on your hands and knees, reach back and grasp your right foot with your left hand (A). Lift the right leg as high as you can, arching your back if possible. Hold for several seconds, breathing normally. Repeat with the left leg. Repetitions: 1 on each side.

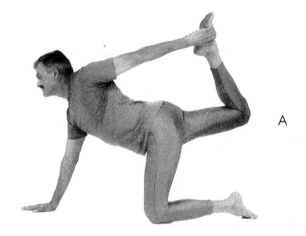

A

Then reach back and grasp the left foot with the left hand (B). Repeat once on the other side.

Keep your balance by staring at one spot on the floor.

Lift the foot as high as possible.

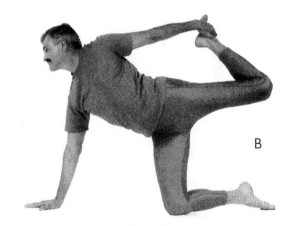

B

Cobra V-Raise (Courses 2 & 3)

- Strengthens legs, upper back, shoulders, and respiratory muscles
- Limbers and strengthens muscles in chest, neck, abdomen, and groin
- Improves function of organs in abdominal region
- Improves reproductive function
- Reduces body fat

This is a combination pose for Course 2 requiring extra strength and stamina. In this exercise only the hands and feet touch the floor. To start from a standing position, lean forward from the hips and "walk" your hands into position out in front. Alternatively, start on your hands and knees. Then breathe out to a count of three as you lift your hips, tucking your head under and pushing your heels toward the floor so that your body looks like an inverted V (A). Hold for a count of three. Then breathe in to a count of three as you lower your hips and arch your back, looking up (B). Try to keep your legs straight and your knees off the floor. Repetitions: 3 to 6.

Variation: For an even greater challenge, try this exercise on your fingertips. This variation strengthens the wrists, forearms, and hands in addition to the above-mentioned benefits.

Breathe deeply, and coordinate breath with movement.
Remember to tuck your head under on the exhalation.

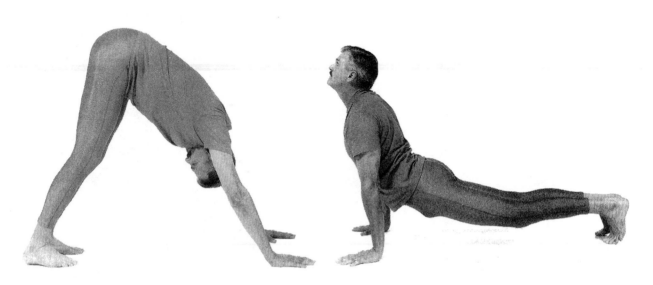

A   B

Forward and Side Plank (Course 3)

- Strengthens wrists, arms, shoulders, and neck
- Improves circulation to entire upper body
- Strengthens back muscles

This is another demanding series for Course 3. This exercise requires strength throughout your body. You will be tempted to hold your breath. However, you must try to let your breath go into its own natural pattern, the Easy Breath pattern, which will be shorter and more forceful—rather like panting. Even though you are using most of your body's strength in this exercise, you should still try to relax your stomach muscles so that your body decides how to breathe. With this physically demanding exercise, you will find that your breath naturally becomes faster and heavier, replenishing your muscles with the oxygen they need.

From the Cobra V-Raise, or from your hands and knees, straighten your legs and position your hips so that your legs and torso make a straight line. Shift your weight to your left hand, then lift your right arm out in front of you, extending the line (A). Look ahead at your middle fingertip and let your breath relax. Hold for a count of three. Repeat with the left arm extended. At first you may not be strong enough to support yourself on one hand. If so, just practice leaning on one hand at a time, back and forth, until your arms gain strength.

Shift your weight back to your left arm and raise your right arm overhead, rotating your body and turning your head to look at your right thumbnail (B). Your body, including both feet, will be twisted sideways. Hold for a count of three, letting your breath relax. Return to the start position, relax, and repeat with the left arm extended.

After practicing these variations separately for a few weeks, you may do them in sequence. Start with the Forward Plank, raising your right arm forward, then immediately bring the arm overhead for the Side Plank. Repeat with the left arm. Repetitions: 1 on each side.

Keep your body straight.
Let the breath relax as much as possible.

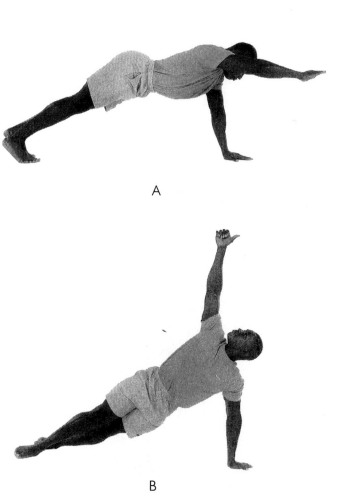

A

B

Hero Pose Variation (Course 2) (*Virasan* Variation)

- Helps strengthen arches of flat feet
- Relieves stiffness in hips, knees, and ankles
- Reduces bloating in stomach and intestines
- Improves respiration
- Improves circulation in entire pelvic region
- Improves reproductive function
- Increases flexibility in lower back and hips
- Reduces body fat

Sit on your feet with rounded arms overhead, one hand on top of the other (A). Breathe in to a count of three as you rise off your feet a few inches, then breathe out to a count of three as you slide to the right (B). Try to keep your knees on the floor as you move. Now breathe in to a count of three as you lift up again and over to the left, breathing out to a count of three as you sit back down. If your legs are not strong enough to do this exercise at first, support yourself lightly with one hand on either side. Try to use your leg muscles as much as possible. Repetitions: 3 to each side. Finish by coming back to the center.

Try to keep your back straight and knees on the floor.
Breathe in as you come up, out as you sit down.

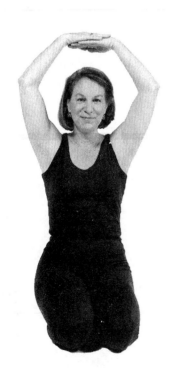

A

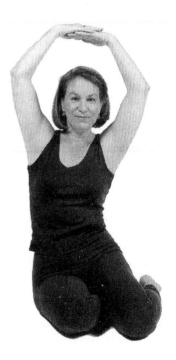

B

Extended Hero Pose (Course 2) (*Virasan* Extension)

- Increases circulation to head
- Improves respiration
- Strengthens and limbers shoulders, ankles, and chest
- Improves posture

Sit on your feet, clasp your hands together low and behind your back, and straighten your arms, locking your elbows (A). Your toes should be just touching and your ankles spread to form a seat for the buttocks. Breathe in to a count of three, then breathe out to a count of three as you bend forward. Raise the arms up and away from the body (B); hold this position for a count of three, then breathe in to a count of three as you come back up to a seated position and relax. Repetitions: 3.

Keep hands clasped and arms straight. Breathe in and out deeply.

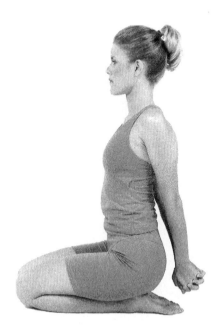

A

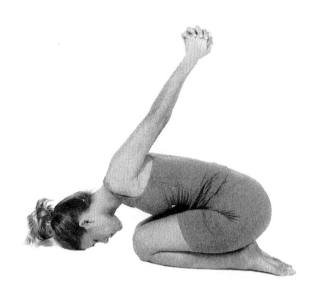

B

Ankle Stretch (Course 2)

- Limbers and strengthens ankles, hips, and knees
- Strengthens abdominal muscles

Sit on your feet, arms at your sides, palms on the floor, breathing normally (A). Gently lift your knees as far as possible while pushing down slightly with your fingers if necessary to intensify the lift (B). Lower your knees and relax. Repetitions: 3.

Breathe normally—don't hold your breath.
Lift your knees high enough to stretch your ankles, but do not strain.

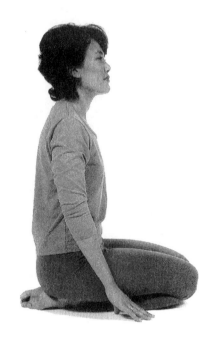

A

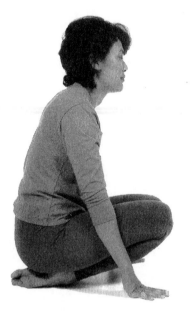

B

Camel Pose (Course 2)

- Limbers entire spine and pelvis
- Opens chest, improving respiration
- Improves circulation in spinal column
- Stretches and strengthens upper and lower thighs and knees

Start in a kneeling position. The first illustration shows a warm-up to this intense stretch. Lean back and grasp your left heel with your left hand (A). Push your hips forward until you feel the muscles being stretched across the pelvis and thighs. Now release, relax, and repeat on the right side. Finally, lean back and grasp both heels. Gently tilt your head back, being careful not to strain your neck. Keep your lips together. Push your hips forward, as if someone has a rope around your waist and is pulling it (B). Hold the position for a few seconds, breathing normally. You should notice your breath moving mostly in the belly area, using the Easy Breath (see p. 50). Repetitions: 1 on each side for the warm-up, just once for the completed pose.

Keep your lips together.
Breathe gently from the belly.

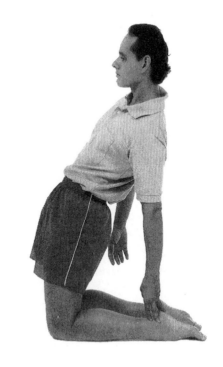

A

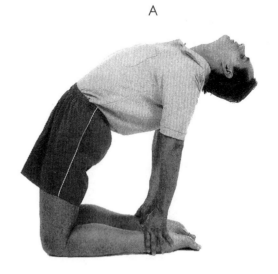

B

Thigh Stretch (Courses 2 & 3) (*Hanumanasan* Preparation)

- Stretches and strengthens abductor muscles of thighs and hips
- Increases circulation to pelvis
- Improves reproductive function

This is an effective exercise for runners because it stretches the hamstrings and groin muscles. Start in a modified lunge, right leg forward, left leg back, resting your left knee on the floor. Your left thigh should be at a 45-degree angle to the floor. Bend your right calf perpendicular to the floor, your fingertips on the floor beside your right foot (A). Breathe in to a count of three as you lean forward, arching your back and looking up (B). Then breathe out and sit back, straightening your right leg and bending your head forward toward your right knee (C). Keep the toes of your right foot pointed straight ahead. Repeat on the left side. Repetitions: 3 each side.

Breathe deeply and smoothly, matching breath with movement.
Do not strain beyond your limits.

A

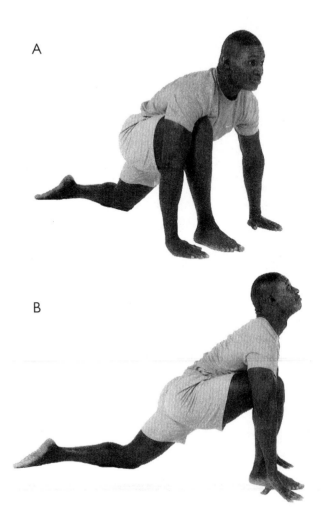

B

C

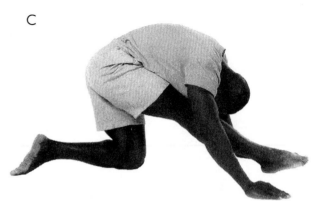

Pigeon Pose (Courses 2 & 3)
(Rajakapotasan)

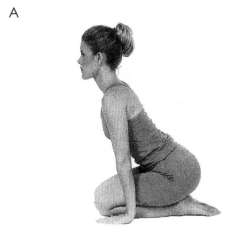

A

- Stretches and strengthens spinal column and all spinal muscles and nerves, especially cervical and sacral vertebrae
- Strengthens and limbers hip joints and groin muscles
- Stimulates metabolic and reproductive glands and organs
- Increases vitality
- Helps relieve impotence
- Strengthens and stretches rib cage and chest

B

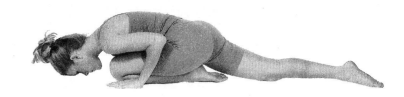

C

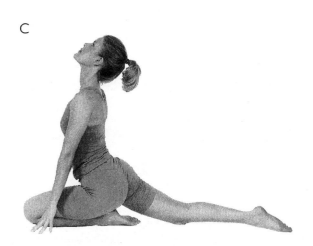

Start by sitting on your heels, with your weight forward (A). Slide your right leg back, keeping the top of your knee on the floor so that your hip and leg do not rotate. You should be sitting directly on top of your left foot. Place your palms next to your left knee and rest your chest on your thigh, forehead to the floor (B). Breathe out completely. Breathe in to a count of three as you lift and curl your torso back as far as possible, curling your head first, then chest and stomach. Come up on your fingertips to further arch the spine (C). Hold for a count of three, then breathe out to a count of three as you lower your torso in reverse order: stomach first, then chest, finally lowering your head after your chest is resting on your thigh again. Repeat on the left side. Repetitions: 3 each side.

Variation: After your hips and knees have become more limber, you may try this exercise with your front leg turned out to the side, so that your front foot is resting on its outer side (D). The back leg must still be placed so that the top of the knee is on the floor.

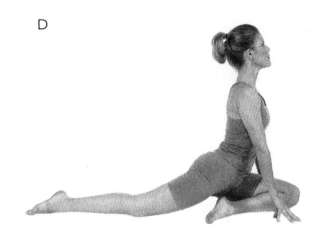

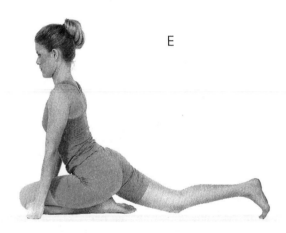

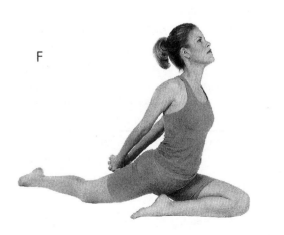

Hold: When the curriculum instructs you to hold the Pigeon Pose, push up on your fists after your third repetition and tuck your toes under in back (E). Fix your gaze on a spot on the floor about 3 feet to the front (do not look up in this hold—keep your neck straight). Relax your stomach muscles, breathe normally, and hold the pose for 10 to 30 seconds.

Variation: Another variation begins with your hands clasped behind your back and arms locked (F). Use the same breath pattern. This variation requires much more back strength.

   Look up and keep your lips together.
   Curl and uncurl your spine.
   Use your hands for support only; use your
      back, not your arm muscles, to hold your
      torso up.

Foot Flaps (Course 1)

- Limber ankles and toes
- Improve mind-body coordination
- Gently stretch sciatic nerve and muscles in backs of legs in preparation for forward-bending poses
- Help relieve varicose veins
- Reduce body fat

A

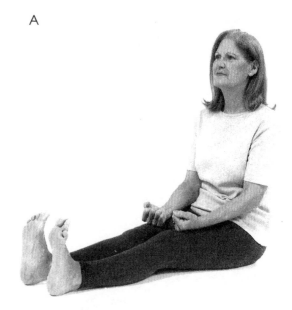

B

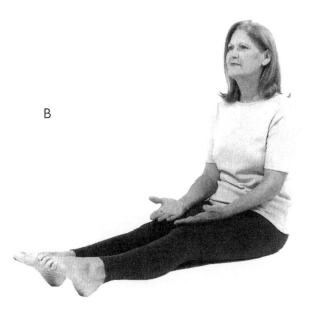

Sit with your legs straight in front of you, heels on the floor. Make fists and rest them on your thighs, palms up, then pull your toes toward your face as far as you can without strain (A). Now open your hands and point your toes away from you (B). Repeat several times. Now open your right hand and make a fist with the left, while pointing your right foot and flexing the left. Alternate and repeat several times. Then, with hands relaxed, rotate your ankles in circles: both one way, then both the other, then opposite ways.

Keep your knees straight.
Breathe normally.

Seated Sun Pose (Courses 1 & 2) *(Paschimottanasan)*

- Strengthens abdominal viscera and diaphragm
- Improves digestive function; may help relieve constipation
- Strengthens nervous system
- Strengthens and stretches legs and spine
- Helps relieve impotence

Sit with your legs extended in front of you, feet flexed, back straight, arms at your sides, palms on the floor (A). Breathe out completely. Breathe in to a count of three as you bring your arms in a wide circle to the sides and over your head. Press your palms together and stretch, looking up at your hands. Hold your breath in for a count of three (B). This position will open the rib cage and improve breathing. Breathe out to a count of three as you bend from the

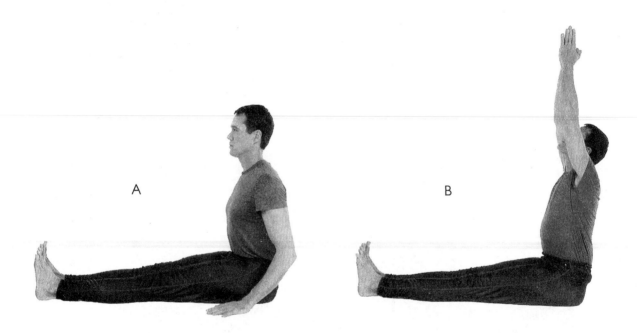

A   B

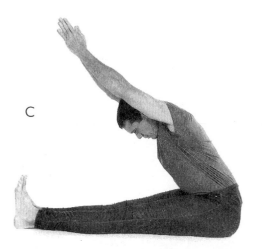

C

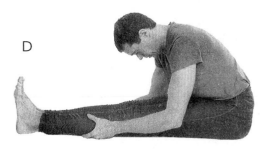

D

Keep your knees straight, feet flexed.

Breathe in and out completely, coordinating breath with movement.

Do not bounce.

Be sure the breath is all the way out at the bottom hold.

hips, tilting your pelvis forward slightly and keeping your head between your arms (C). Keep your feet flexed and knees straight. Bend forward from the waist as far as you comfortably can and grasp underneath your legs firmly at the knees, calves, or ankles. Hold your breath out for a count of three as you gently pull your upper body down toward your legs, bending your elbows (D). Do not bounce or strain. If you cannot bend your elbows, grab your legs farther up until you can. Then breathe in to a count of three as you straighten, bringing your arms to the sides and up in a wide circle, breathing in all the way to the top. Press your palms together, stretch up, and look up at your hands. Hold your breath in for a count of three. Then breathe out to a count of three as you lower your arms slowly to your sides and relax. If you have a weak back, you can do this exercise seated with your back against the wall.

If you can reach your toes and still bend your elbows easily, you are already quite limber in your hips and the backs of your legs. Wrap your fingers around your big toes, as shown (E and F). This position completes a nerve circuit in your body and will enhance the effectiveness of the exercise.

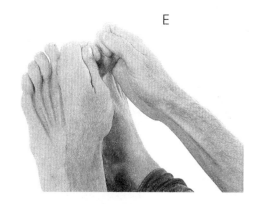

E

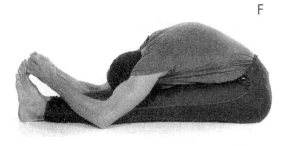

F

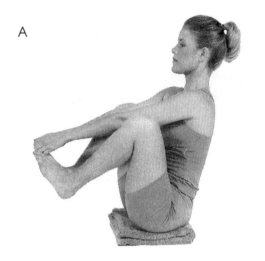

A

Sun Pose Balance (Course 2)
(*Paschimottanasan* Variation)

- Strengthens abdominal muscles
- Increases circulation in torso
- Strengthens hip joints and legs
- Helps develop mental stability

Begin in à seated position. Grasp your ankles or toes (A). Then lean back a little and find your center of balance. Slowly try to straighten your legs (B and C). Hold the position for several seconds, breathing normally. You may have to support yourself with a folded blanket or towel under your buttocks.

Find your balance before straightening your
  legs.
Don't hold your breath.

B

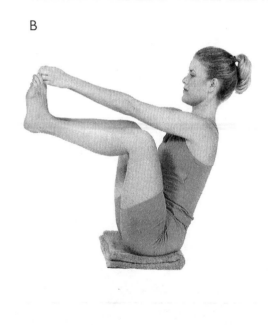

C

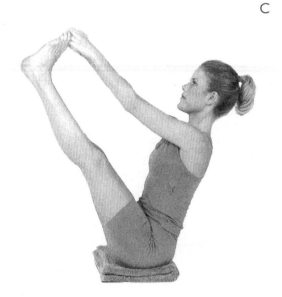

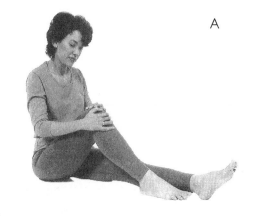

A

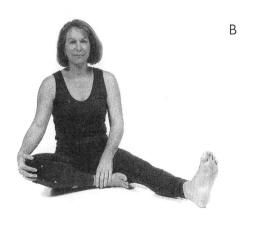

B

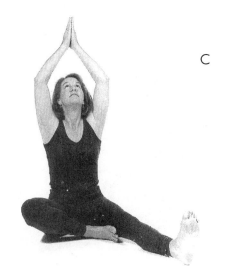

C

Alternate Seated Sun Pose (Courses 1, 2, & 3) (*Paschimottanasan*)

- Same overall benefits as Seated Sun Pose
- Improves hip and knee limberness

Sit with your legs extended in front of you. Bend your right knee and massage it for several seconds to warm and relax the joint (A). Supporting the knee with your hands, gently lower it to the floor, and with your left hand place the sole of your right foot against the inside of your left thigh as high as possible (B). Flex the toes of your outstretched left leg. Sit up straight, arms at your sides, and exhale completely. Breathe in to a count of three as you bring your arms in a wide circle to the sides and overhead. Press your palms together, stretch up, looking up at your hands, and hold your breath in for a count of three (C). Breathe out to a count of three as you bend forward from the hips, keeping your head between your arms. Bend as far as you can without strain. Grasp your left leg with both hands, bend your elbows, and pull your upper body toward your leg (D). Your breath should be completely out. Hold for a count of three, then breathe in to a count of three as you bring your arms in a wide circle over-

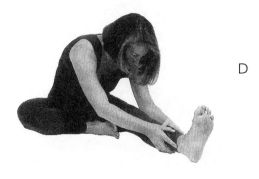

D

head. Press your palms together, stretch and look up, hold for a count of three, then relax and breathe out to a count of three as you bring your arms back down to the sides. Repeat with your right leg extended. Repetitions: 3 times to each side.

Just as in the Seated Sun Pose, try to reach your toes when you bend forward. Eventually, you may be able to grasp your big toe with both hands as you pull your upper body toward your outstretched leg.

After your hip joints become more limber, you may try this exercise with your foot resting on top of the opposite thigh. However, if you can't hold this position without your knee coming more than 3 or 4 inches off the floor, you're not ready for it. Instead, practice the Limber Hips exercise (following) often. If you put your foot on top of your thigh, be sure to rest the whole foot, not just the toes, on the thigh.

> Bend from the hips, not the waist.
> Breathe slowly and completely, matching
>   breath with movement.
> Keep the toes on your outstretched leg flexed.

Limber Hips (Course 1)

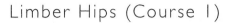

⬤ Limbers hip and knee joints

This exercise helps prepare you for a more comfortable seated position. After the Alternate Seated Sun Pose, support your bent knee, pick up your left foot, and place the foot on top of your outstretched right leg (A). Lean back on your right hand. With your left hand, gently press down on the bent left knee and release several times. Repeat with the right leg. This is an exercise you can do at various times of the day to loosen the knee and hip joints.

When your hips and knees have become more limber, pick up the knee and foot as illustrated and pull the foot close to your chest (B). Then move the foot to one ear (as if it were a telephone!) and then the other.

> Breathe normally.
> Press down and pull up gently on the bent knee.

A

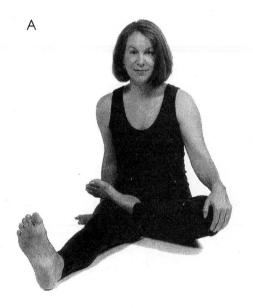

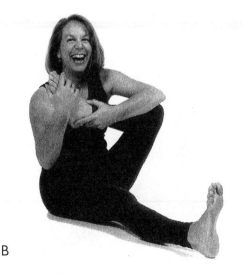

B

Easy Spine Twist (Course I)

- Gently limbers spine in preparation for full Spine Twist
- Helps improves digestion and eyesight
- Strengthens nervous system

Sit in a comfortable cross-legged position. Place your right hand on the floor behind your right hip, straighten your arm, and place your left hand on the outside of your right knee. Straighten your back and look forward. Breathe in to a count of three. Then breathe out to a count of three as you twist toward the right, keeping your head straight, following a horizontal line at eye level as far as you can (A). Hold the position for a count of three, then release and breathe in to a count of three as you come back around to the front. Repeat to the left.

Variation: Straighten your left leg and bend your right leg, lifting the right foot over to the opposite side of the left leg near the knee. With your left hand, reach under the lifted knee and grasp your thigh on the outside. You can pull with this hand to twist further. Place your right hand on the floor behind your hip. Straighten your back (straightening your right arm will help) and look forward, breathing in to a count of three. Breathe out to a count of three as you twist to the right as far as possible, keeping your head straight, following a horizontal line at eye level as far as you can, then fixing your gaze on a spot at eye level on the wall (B). Hold for a count of three, then release. Repeat with the left leg bent.

In any lateral twist to the spine, it is important to keep your back and head erect. If you slouch or tuck your chin to your chest before twisting, you will end up with a spiral instead of a side twist.

Keep your spine and head erect.
Breathe normally while holding the pose.
Exert a little pull with the forward hand to increase the twist.

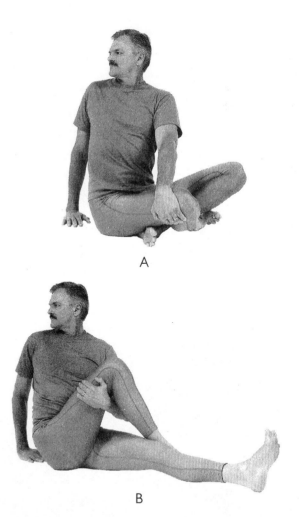

A

B

Spine Twist (Courses 1, 2, & 3)
(Ardha Matsyendrasan)

- Helps relieve chronic constipation
- Helps relieve urinary, bladder, and prostate difficulties
- Strengthens respiratory muscles
- Improves digestion
- Stimulates spinal column nerves
- Limbers hips, spine, and shoulders

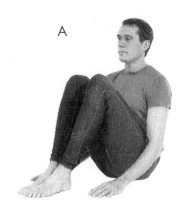

A

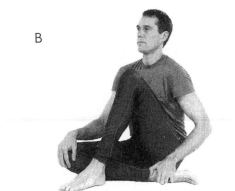

B

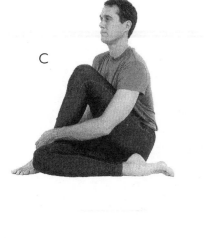

C

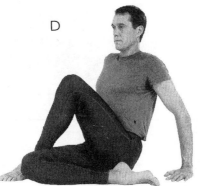

D

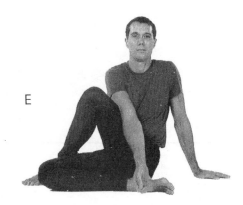

E

Start with both legs bent in front (A). Weave your right leg under the left, so the right knee rests on the floor and the right foot is curled beside the left hip (B). Place your left foot on the outside of your right knee (C). Always twist toward the raised leg, but first, ensure that your spine is straight with this check: Lean back on both hands and arch your spine slightly, keeping your head forward so as not to strain your neck (D). Now straighten your spine up and twist to the left, lifting your rib cage and placing both hands on the floor beside your right foot (E). Your right arm should be entirely on the outside of your raised (left) leg. Note: If you have trouble with this step, try this instead: Reach under the lifted left leg with your right arm and hold on to the outside of your left thigh with your right hand as in the Easy Spine Twist (F). Continue with the instructions that follow in the next paragraph. Now bend your right arm, lift your rib cage and, with your right elbow, gently push your left knee back and forth a few times. Now push it back as far as it will go, straighten your arm, and grasp your pant leg, your right knee, or your left ankle (G). The important thing is to keep that right arm on the outside of your left knee. That arm is a lever that twists the right side of your body—especially the upper torso—as far to the left as possible.

Now place your left hand behind you at the base of your spine, straightening your arm and pointing your fingers in toward your body. Keep your hand as close to your back as possible (H). If your hand is too far away from you, your back will curve into a slouch and your spine will not achieve a good lateral stretch. The lower back area is especially likely to slouch, so before you twist, lift your rib cage and straighten your lower back by pushing your pelvis slightly forward and straightening your support arm. Straighten your spine, look forward, and breathe in to a count of three. Breathe out to a count. of three as you twist to the left, keeping your head erect and eyes focused on a spot at eye level as far to the left as you can see comfortably. Hold the position with the breath out for a count of three. Then release and breathe in to a count of three as you come back forward. Switch sides. Repetitions: 1 each side.

Keep your spine and head erect.
Focus your eyes on one spot.

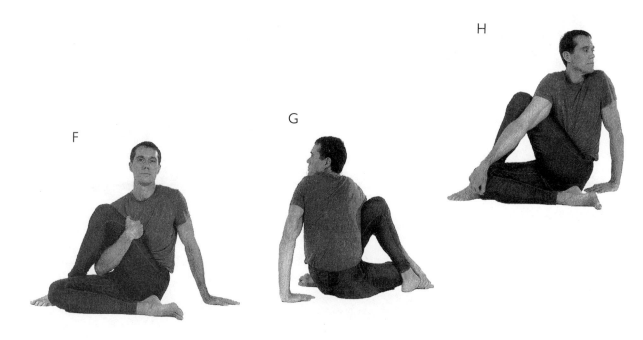

Diamond Pose Warm-up (Courses 1 & 2) (Bhadrasan)

- Strengthens and limbers hip joints
- Helps relieve urinary difficulties
- Reduces susceptibility to hernia
- Helps prostate difficulties
- Helps relieve impotence

Sit with the soles of your feet together about a foot from your body and let your knees fall toward the floor as far as possible. Grasp your ankles with both hands (A). Breathe in to a count of three as you straighten your spine, then breathe out to a count of three as you lean forward, pressing down on your thighs with your elbows (B). As you breathe in to a count of three and straighten up, pull your feet a little closer to your body. Breathe out to a count of three as you bend forward again. Repeat once more for a total of 3.

Breathe deeply.

Grab your ankles with your hands and press down with your elbows.

Do not strain. Hip and groin muscles take a fair amount of time to stretch out, so be patient.

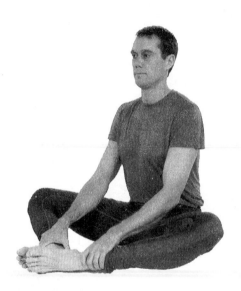

A

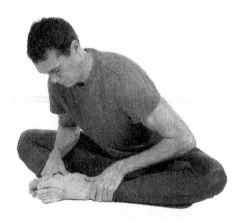

B

Diamond Pose (Courses 1, 2, & 3)
(Shiva Shaktiasan)

- Strengthens nervous system
- Strengthens and stretches sciatic nerves
- Improves digestion
- Strengthens and limbers hip joints
- Limbers lower back

Place the soles of your feet together about a foot from your body. Lace your fingers around your toes (C). Straighten your spine and breathe in to a count of three. Then breathe out to a count of three as you bend forward from the hips as far as you can without strain, letting your elbows fall outside your knees (D). Hold for a count of three. Breathe in to a count of three as you straighten up. With practice, you'll be able to touch your forehead to your big toes. Repetitions: 3.

Keep your spine straight.
Clasp your toes.
Keep your elbows outside your legs.

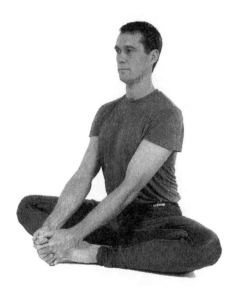

C

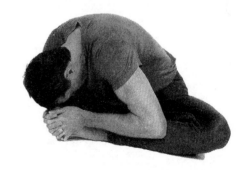

D

Hero Pose (Courses 2 & 3)
(*Virasan*)

- Stretches nerves and muscles of spinal column
- Stretches lower back
- Stretches and strengthens hips, knees, and ankles
- Stretches sciatic nerves and thigh muscles

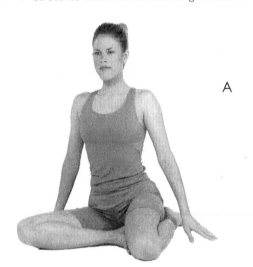

A

tween your knees. Hold for a count of three, then breathe in to a count of three as you straighten up. With the next exhalation, bring your head in a little farther toward the left knee. On the third repetition, hold the downward position, breathing gently (B). Hold for several seconds, then release and repeat on the opposite side. Repetitions: 1 on each side.

When you become more limber, you may put your right foot on top of your left thigh (the whole foot, not just the toes), bringing your knees a little closer together (C). Repeat on the opposite side. This variation greatly increases the stretch on the hip joints and knees.

Relax your hips and legs.
Curl your toes around the hip.

B

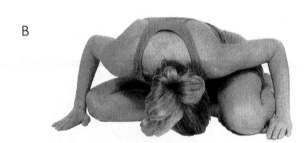

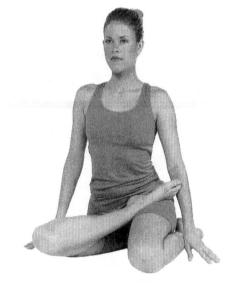

C

Start in a seated position with your right foot against the inside of your left thigh and your left foot drawn close to but not under the left buttock (A). Place your hands on the floor alongside each knee, straighten your back, breathe in to a count of three, then breathe out to a count of three as you bend forward, aiming your head at the midpoint be-

Side Stretch (Course 3)

- Stretches side and intercostal muscles
- Limbers vertebrae
- Relieves tension in upper back and shoulders

Sit in a comfortable cross-legged position with arms at your sides. Breathe normally throughout the exercise. Shift your weight to the right, supporting yourself with your right hand or elbow, and bring your left arm over your head in a plane with your body (A). Let the weight of your arm stretch the muscles along your left side. Bend your spine as far sideways as it will go without straining. Hang there for several seconds, then switch sides. Next, reverse the position of your feet and repeat.

Keep your upper arm in a plane with the body.
Breathe normally.
Let the weight of your arm do the stretching.

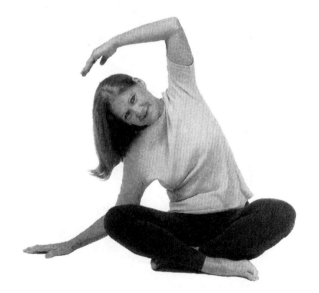

A

Intense Floor Stretch (Course 1)
(Uttihitasan)

- Stretches muscles of torso and hips
- Expands and stretches muscles of rib cage
- Stretches muscles along spine
- Relieves back strain

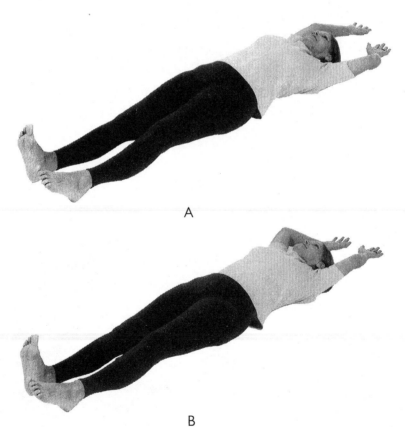

A

B

Start by lying down with both arms resting on the floor over your head. Reach up with your right hand and push down with your left foot (A). Repeat on the opposite side. Then stretch the same sides: left hand and left foot; right hand and right foot (B).

Keep your feet flexed.
Breathe normally.

Knee Squeeze (Courses 1, 2, & 3) (*Pavanamuktasan*)

- Relieves gas, bloated sensation, and heartburn
- Helps relieve constipation
- Increases circulation in head and neck
- Reduces body fat
- Relieves lower back tension
- Strengthens abdominal muscles

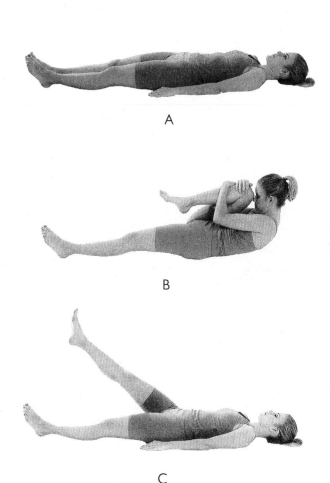

Lie flat on your back with arms at your sides (A). Breathe in to a count of three as you raise your right knee to your chest and your forehead to your knee. Make sure your lungs are full, wrap your arms around your knee, and hold your breath in for a count of three as you squeeze your knee to your chest (B). Breathe out to a count of three as you slowly relax, straightening your leg (C) until it rests on the floor. Repeat with your left leg. Repetitions: 3 on each side, alternating sides. Then rest a moment, breathing gently.

Variation: Now try lifting both legs (D). In this variation it is important to breathe in to a count of three first, then hold your breath in for a count of three while you squeeze. If you try to breathe in and lift at the same time, you will not get a complete lungful of air because you will be tightening your stomach muscles to help lift your legs. Relax and breathe out. Repetitions: 3.

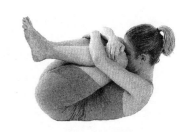

Hold a full lungful of air in as you squeeze.
In the Double Knee Squeeze, breathe in first and hold your breath while you lift both knees to your chest.
Hold the squeeze only a few seconds to start.

The Walk (Courses 2 & 3)

- Reduces body fat
- Strengthens legs
- Helps relieve constipation
- Strengthens lower back

Lie flat, arms at your sides, palms down. Bend your legs, then raise and straighten them so they are pointing toward the ceiling, forming a 90-degree angle with your body. Breathing normally, start "walking" back and forth, keeping your legs straight and your feet flexed (A). Continue this motion for 10 to 30 seconds, then bend your knees and slowly lower your legs to the floor.

Keep your legs straight.
Keep your feet flexed.
Breathe normally.

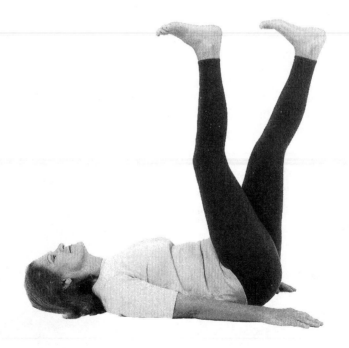

A

Alternate Toe Touch (Course 2)
(Supta Padangusthasan)

- Tones, strengthens, and stretches muscles in legs and hips
- Helps relieve sciatica
- Strengthens nerves and muscles in hips and pelvis
- Strengthens lower back

Lie on your back with your arms overhead. Breathe in to a count of three as you raise your left leg and left arm simultaneously (A). Keep your left foot flexed, your shoulders and head on the floor, and your right leg straight. If you cannot touch your toes, bring your hand and foot as close together as possible. Hold for a count of three, then relax and breathe out to a count of three as you lower your leg and arm. Repeat on the right side. Repetitions: 3 on each side.

Variation: With the same breath pattern, lift opposite arm and leg (B). Repetitions: 3 on each side.

Keep your shoulders and head on the floor.
Keep both legs straight.
Match breath with movement.

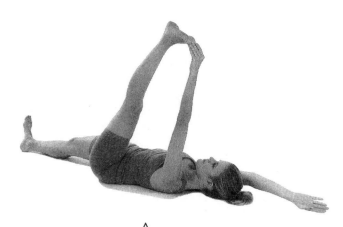

A

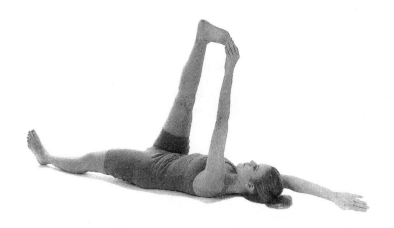

B

Easy Fish Pose (Course 2)
(*Matsyasan* Variation)

- Fully expands chest for improved breathing and circulation
- Improves flexibility in neck and lower back
- Helps remove calcium deposits from spinal column
- Helps relieve illnesses of throat
- Improves functioning of thyroid
- Strengthens eyesight
- Tones facial and throat muscles

A

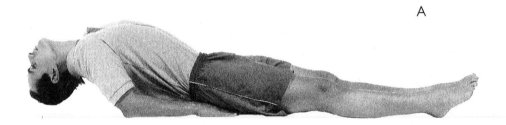

Do not do this exercise if you have neck problems. Lie flat on your back and slide your hands just under your thighs. Now use your arms and back muscles to lift your body, from the waist up, off the floor. Arch your back and neck so that the top of your head rests on the floor (A). Keep your lips together and jut your lower jaw forward. Keep your eyes open and look at the floor, breathing gently. Hold this position for several seconds, then release and lower your torso to the floor. Relax.

As you rise from the prone position, come up on one elbow first, then slide the other hand behind you, as shown (B), and push yourself up. This intermediary step will keep you from tensing your back muscles and possibly straining your back when you lift.

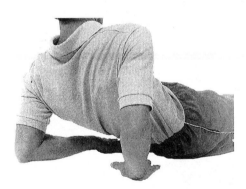

B

Fish Pose (Course 2)
(Matsyasan)

After you have been practicing for several months, you may wish to try the full Fish Pose. Start in a seated position with feet separated so your hips rest on the floor, keeping your knees as close together as possible. Lean back on your elbows. Usually this is as far as most students can go until the thigh and groin muscles loosen up more. Keep practicing this intermediary step and eventually you will be able to take the full position as shown (C).

Keep your lips and teeth together.
Keep your eyes open.
Let the breath relax into the belly.

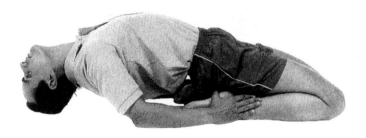

C

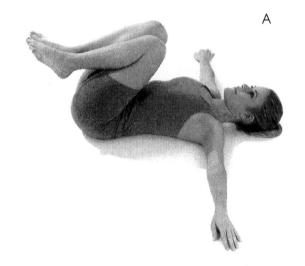

A

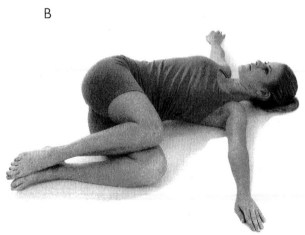

B

feet off the floor as if you were going to do a Double Knee Squeeze (A). This is your start position. Breathe in to a count of three as you slowly swing your legs toward the floor to the left, keeping your knees bent (B). If you wish, and if you do not have neck problems, you may turn your head to the right to extend the stretch higher up your torso. Breathe out to a count of three as you slowly raise your legs back to the start position. Then breathe in to a count of three as you lower them to the right. Breathe out to a count of three and return to the center. Be sure to keep your shoulders and arms on the floor at all times. Repetitions: 3 on each side.

Variation: After doing this exercise for several weeks, you may move on to this variation. Keep the same start position, but as you lower your legs to the side, breathing in to a count of three, straighten them so that they are parallel to your outstretched arm (C). Repetitions: 3 on each side.

Keep your shoulders and arms on the floor. Breathe deeply and slowly, matching breath with movement.

Pelvic Twist (Course 1)
(Jathara Parivarthanasan)

- Improves function of liver, spleen, pancreas, stomach, kidneys, and intestines
- Reduces body fat
- Strengthens lower back and hips

Do not do this exercise if you have lower back problems. Lie on your back with your arms extended to the sides, palms down. Lift your legs and

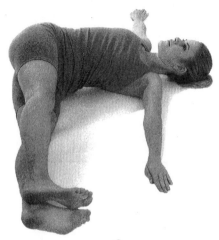

C

Easy Bridge (Courses 1, 2, & 3)

- Improves function of thyroid and parathyroid glands, thereby helping improve function of entire endocrine system
- Eases back pain and fatigue
- Increases circulation to head and face, improving complexion and eyesight
- Helps manage hypertension
- Increases metabolism

Lie on your back with knees bent, feet a few inches apart and as close to your buttocks as possible. Arms are at your sides and palms down (A). Breathe out completely, and relax your shoulders, neck, and head. Breathe in to a count of three as you raise your hips off the floor as if there were a rope tied around your waist pulling you up. Arch your back, keeping your shoulders on the floor (B). Your lungs should be filled in the arched position. Hold for a count of three. Now breathe out to a count of three as you slowly lower your hips to the floor. Be sure not to turn your head in this position. Repetitions: 3. If you can reach your ankles easily, you may do this exercise holding on to your ankles as shown (C).

Keep your shoulders and neck relaxed.
Place your feet as close to your body as possible.

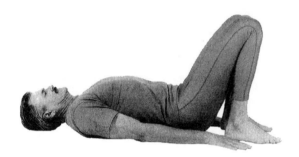

A

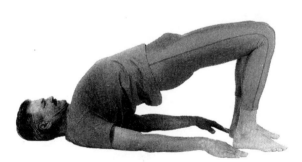

B

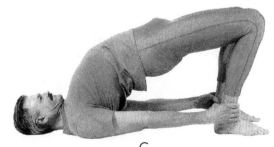

C

Easy Sit-up (Courses 2 & 3)

- Strengthens abdominal muscles and upper back
- Relieves stomach and breath tension
- Massages internal organs

Lie on your back with your knees bent, feet flat on the floor and a comfortable distance apart. With arms straight, place your hands on your thighs, fingers a few inches from your knees (A). Now breathe in to a count of three until your lungs are about one-half full, and hold your breath to a count of three as you lift your head and upper body and slide your hands up to your knees (B). Hold for a count of three, then relax and breathe out to a count of three. Repetitions: 3.

Keep your arms straight.
Hold breath in as you lift.

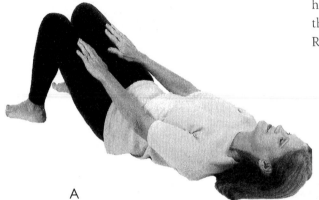

A

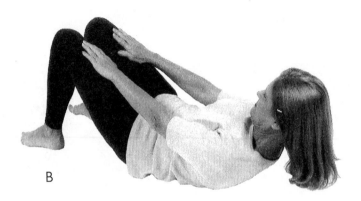

B

Neck Curl (Courses 2 & 3)

- Strengthens stomach and upper back
- Relieves breath and stomach tension

Similar to the Easy Sit-up, this exercise is a little easier on the neck for those with neck problems. Lie on your back, with your knees bent and feet a comfortable distance apart. Place your hands on your upper back and shoulders, spreading your fingers to support your neck (A). Alternatively, cross your arms on your chest, holding opposite shoulders. Breathe in to a count of three to one-half capacity, then hold your breath in for a count of three and lift, using your back and stomach muscles (B). Do not strain. Relax and breathe out to a count of three. Repetitions: 3.

Hold breath in while lifting.
Support your neck.

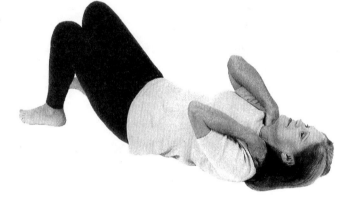

A

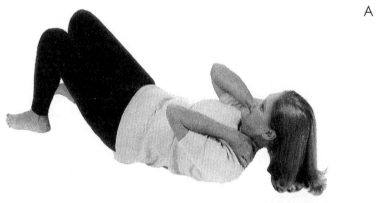

B

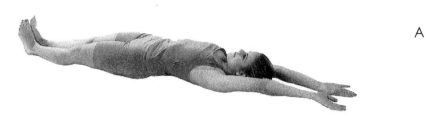

A

Big Sit-up (Courses 2 & 3)
(Supta Padangusthasan)

- Strengthens abdominal viscera and all abdominal and thigh muscles
- Improves balance and concentration
- Strengthens legs
- Helps relieve constipation and difficulties of urinary tract

This is the most challenging of the sit-up exercises. Lie flat on your back with arms extended overhead (A). Breathe in to a count of three to about one-half capacity, then hold your breath in as you bring fingers and toes together, your torso and legs forming a V. Balancing on the end of your spine, try to touch your toes (B) and hold for a count of three. Then breathe out to a count of three as you lower. Repetitions: 3 to 6.

Keep your legs straight.
Hold breath in as you raise.
Breathe shallowly.

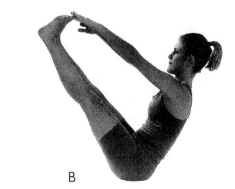

B

Alternate Big Sit-up (Course 3)

- Strengthens transverse abdominal muscles
- Strengthens lower back and shoulders
- Limbers and strengthens hip joints

Lie on your back with arms at your sides. Breathe in to a count of three, to about one-half capacity, hold your breath in, then lift your right arm, your torso, and your left leg, leaning on your left elbow (C). Keep your right foot flexed. Touch your toes if possible, hold your breath for a count of three, then breathe out and return to the start position. Repeat on the opposite side. Repetitions: 3 to 6 each side, alternating.

Keep your legs and arms straight.
Hold breath in as you lift.
Lean on the opposite elbow for support.

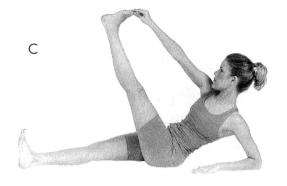

C

The Roll (Course 1)

● Helps make spine flexible and limber in preparation for Shoulder Stand

If you are practicing on a hard surface, use your blanket or mat to protect your back. Sit with knees drawn up to your chest, head down, back rounded, and arms clasped around your knees (A). Holding this position, roll backward on your spine (B), then roll up to a seated position. Be sure to give yourself enough momentum. If you find that your back is too stiff to stay rounded, you can place your hands on the floor next to your body and push off. Roll back and forth several times. Practice this exercise for a few weeks before attempting the Shoulder Stand.

Keep your chin tucked in.
Round your back as much as possible.

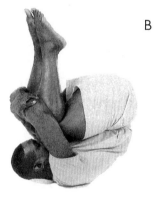

B

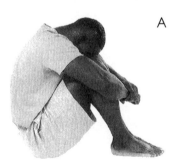

A

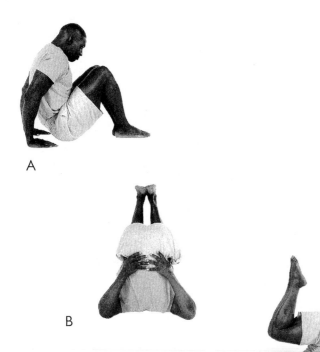

A

B

C

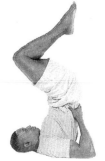

D

This pose should not be done by people with high blood pressure, heart disease, or neck problems without specific permission from your doctor. Do not do this exercise if you have sinus problems or head congestion from a cold or the flu.

The start position is the same as for The Roll, but place your hands on the floor at your sides and slightly back, fingers pointing forward. (A). Roll back onto your shoulders, keeping your knees bent and supporting your back with your hands (B). Be sure to support your back with your hands throughout the exercise. Your knees should touch your fore-

Shoulder Stand (Courses 1, 2, & 3) (Sarvangasan)

- Tones entire endocrine system through stimulation of thyroid and parathyroid glands
- Increases sluggish metabolism
- Enhances function of all vital organs
- Improves reproductive function
- Helps relieve many respiratory difficulties
- Improves eyesight
- Improves circulation
- Relaxes entire nervous system
- Relieves constipation
- Helps prevent yeast infections
- Removes fatigue, makes mind bright and clear

head. Relax your shoulders and head. If you are comfortable, start to lift your knees away from your forehead until your thighs are parallel to the floor (C). Continue straightening your legs while supporting your back with your hands (D). At first, extend your legs behind you; in this position your weight will be more on your upper back, between the shoulder blades, than on your neck (E). Practice this Half Shoulder Stand for several days before going on to the completed pose.

In the completed pose (F), try to straighten your legs perpendicular to the floor. Toes may be relaxed or slightly pointed. You will notice that you can straighten your body more by bringing your hands farther down your back toward the floor and pressing gently while supporting. Your weight is now on the back of your neck. Hold the position, breathing gently, for several seconds. Fix your gaze on the space between your big toes; your feet should be touching. If your eyes get tired, close them for a mo-

pushing off from a chair (G) or a wall (H) until your back and arms develop the proper supportive strength.

Support your back at all times.
Straighten your legs slowly.
Breathe normally.
Relax as much as possible.

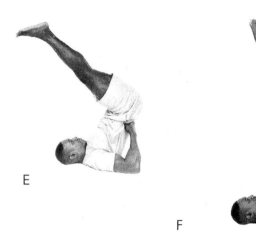

E

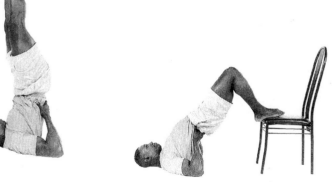

F

G

ment. In the beginning, hold this pose for only 10 to 15 seconds. Do not turn your head.

To come out of the Shoulder Stand safely, bend your knees and bring them to your forehead. Then cross your ankles and gently roll forward all the way, so that your legs fall apart into a cross-legged position and your head is bent forward. This will prevent blood rushing out of your head too quickly. Remain in this position for several seconds.

If you have difficulty lifting your legs, you may lack strength in your arms and back. If so, practice

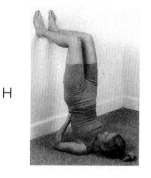

H

Plow Pose (Courses 1, 2, & 3) (Halasan)

- Stimulates thyroid and parathyroid glands, improving function of entire endocrine system
- Gives a complete stretch to spinal cord, nerves, and muscles, and muscles and nerves of legs
- Relieves constipation, lumbago, and rheumatism
- Reduces body fat
- Relieves enlargement of liver and spleen
- Improves posture and suppleness of spine
- Stretches arteries and veins, making them more supple, elastic, and strong

The Plow Pose intensifies the stretch to the spine. The start position is the same as for the Shoulder Stand. Roll back, knees to your forehead, but instead of lifting your legs up, slowly straighten them and lower your toes toward the floor (A). Keep supporting your back with your hands. Notice that your toes are tucked under, pointing toward your head, and your heels are pushing away from your body, increasing the stretch on the backs of your legs. If you cannot reach the floor with your toes and are afraid of injury by rolling back too far on your neck, practice this position either with a chair (B) or by walking your feet down the wall.

When you get into position, you can release the back support and extend your arms, palms down (C). Hold the position for several seconds, breathing gently. Be sure to avoid this position and the Shoulder Stand if you have a head cold or nasal congestion. A headache after doing this exercise is an indication that you are putting too much strain on

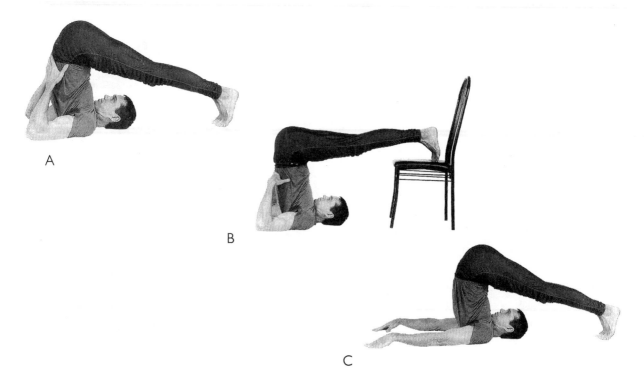

A

B

C

the muscles and nerves, especially in the back of your neck. Proceed more cautiously.

When you have gained flexibility, stamina, and assurance in this pose, you may try some of the variations. Bring your arms overhead and reach for your big toes (D). Press your heels toward the floor as far as possible. Next, lower your knees so that they rest on the floor beside your ears. Hold on to your feet with both hands (E). Now straighten your legs, grab your big toes, and spread your legs as far as possible (F). Bring your legs back together, lift them off the floor until you are balanced, then straighten your arms slowly up toward the ceiling, resting on your shoulders and neck (G). This variation brings a beautiful complexion and clarity of mind.

To come out of the Plow Pose, bring your knees to your forehead, support your back with your hands, and slowly roll forward, bending your head over your crossed legs as you did after the Shoulder Stand. Always use common sense when practicing these asans; never strain past your physical limitations. Yoga is a nonviolent practice.

Keep your legs straight and shoulders relaxed.
Breathe gently.
Do not exceed your limits.

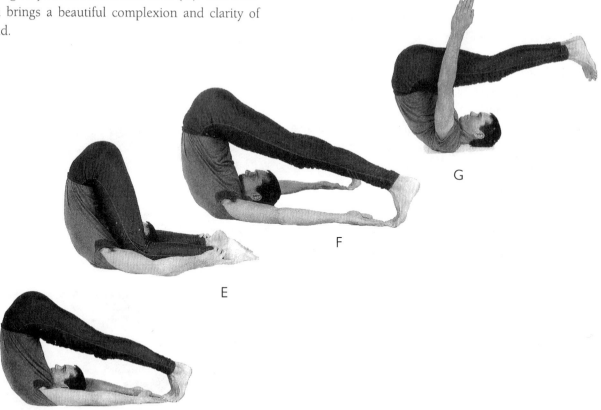

G

F

E

D

Easy Plow Breath (Course 3)

- Relieves tension in breath and midsection
- Strengthens abdominal, lower back, and leg muscles
- Stimulates functioning of internal organs

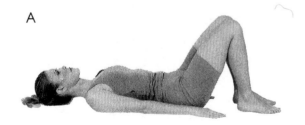

A

Begin by lying on your back, with knees bent and feet flat on the floor. Arms are at your sides, palms down (A). Breathe in fully to a count of three, then breathe out to a count of three as you straighten your legs up (B) and bring them over your head until your toes are several inches above the floor (C). You will need to give yourself some momentum, using your arms, to lift your legs up and over. Notice that bringing your legs over your head has the effect of naturally pushing your breath out in an exhalation. Now start to breathe in to a count of three as you lower your legs. When your hips touch the floor, bend your knees and plant your feet flat on the floor as in the start position (A). Your breath should be completely in at this point. Immediately breathe out to a count of three as you bring your legs up straight again and over your head, repeating the first movement with the exhalation. Repetitions: 3 to 6.

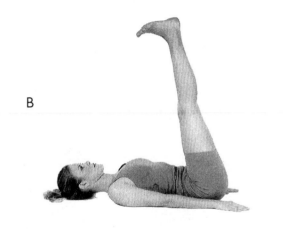

B

Use your arms only to augment your back muscles.

Keep your legs straight when lifting them over your head.

Breathe out when your legs go over your head; breathe in when they come back down to the floor.

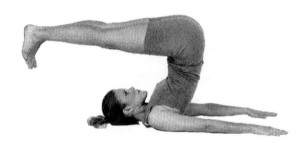

C

Plow Breath (Course 3)

- Relieves tension in breath and midsection
- Strengthens abdominal, lower back, and leg muscles
- Stimulates function of internal organs

This is a movement similar to the previous exercise, but with legs straight. Start lying on your back with arms at your sides, palms down (A). Breathe in to a count of three, hold your breath in, and lift your legs, keeping them straight (B). As your legs swing through perpendicular, start breathing out to a count of three. Your legs going over your head will force the breath out further. Continue lowering your legs until they touch the floor over your head, as in the Plow Pose (C). Now start breathing in as you lift your legs up and back down. Try not to touch the floor in front with your heels but lift your legs in another repetition right away. Repetitions: 3 to 6.

Keep your legs straight.
Breathe out as your legs go over your head; breathe in as they come back down to the floor.
Try to let the motion of your body control your breath.

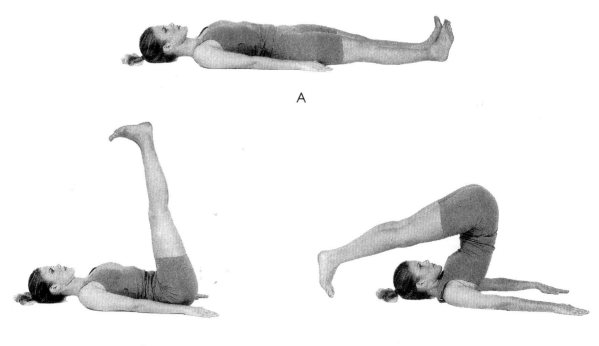

A

B

C

Back Strengtheners
(Courses 1 & 2)

- Strengthens all back muscles and entire spinal column
- Increases abdominal pressure and circulation, which can improve digestion and functioning of vital organs
- Encourages weight loss

Lie on your stomach on the floor, with arms stretched over your head (A). Bend your left arm at the elbow and rest your forehead on your left hand, palm down. Your right arm remains outstretched (B). If you have upper back problems, bend both arms. Breathe out. Now breathe in and count to three as you lift your right arm and your head. Look up. Hold for a count of three, then breathe out and lower. Switch sides. Repetitions: 3 each side, alternating.

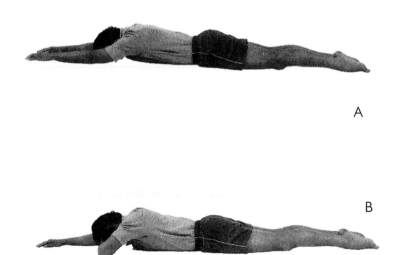

A

B

After a few days of practicing this variation, go on to the next. Get into the same position (B), with your forehead resting on your left hand. This time, raise your right arm, head, and left leg while breathing in and counting to three (C). Look up and hold for a count of three. Breathe out and count to three as you relax. Repeat with opposite limbs. Later you can straighten both arms (D). Repetitions: 3 each side, alternating.

The final back strengtheners involve lifting the arms and legs separately. Start with arms stretched over your head, forehead to the floor (A). Breathe out. Now breathe in and count to three as you lift both arms and your head (E). Hold for a count of three, then breathe out and relax. Repetitions: 3. Then try lifting just your legs (F). Repetitions: 3.

Keep your legs and arms straight as they are lifted.

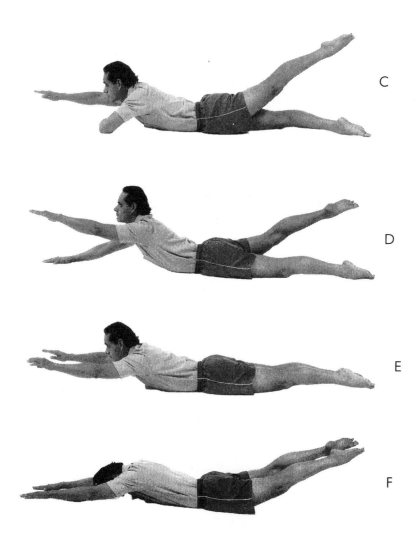

C

D

E

F

Boat Pose (Courses 1 & 2)
(Poorva Navasan)

- Strengthens all back muscles and entire spinal column
- Increases abdominal pressure, which improves digestion and functioning of vital organs

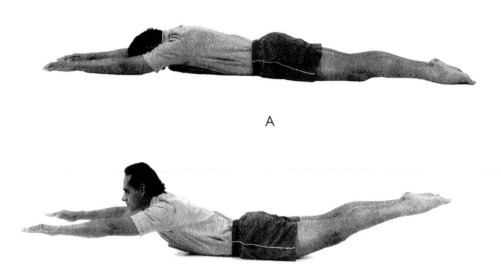

A

B

Lie on your stomach, forehead to the floor, arms stretched over your head (A). Breathe out to a count of three. Then breathe in to a count of three and lift your arms, head, and legs as high as possible (B). Look up, hold for a count of three, then breathe out to a count of three as you relax. Repetitions: 3.

Keep your legs and arms straight.

Airplane Series (Course 2)

- Strengthens entire back and spinal column
- Improves function of vital organs
- Limbers spinal column and shoulder joints
- Strengthens arms, shoulders, hips, and thighs
- Expands rib cage, improving respiration

Try this more challenging series after you have become proficient with the Back Strengtheners and Boat Pose. Lie on your stomach with arms stretched over your head (A). Breathe in to a count of three as you lift arms, head, and legs (B). Breathe out to a count of three as you relax, but swing your arms out to the sides, perpendicular to your body (C). Relax completely in this position. Now breathe in to a

A

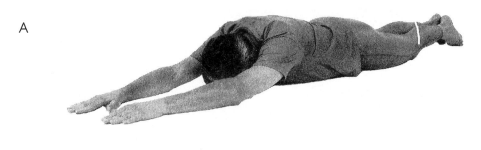

B

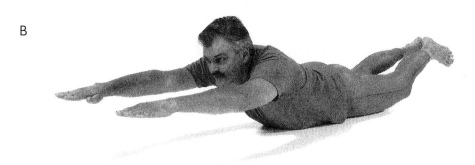

C

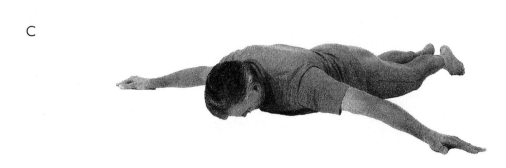

D

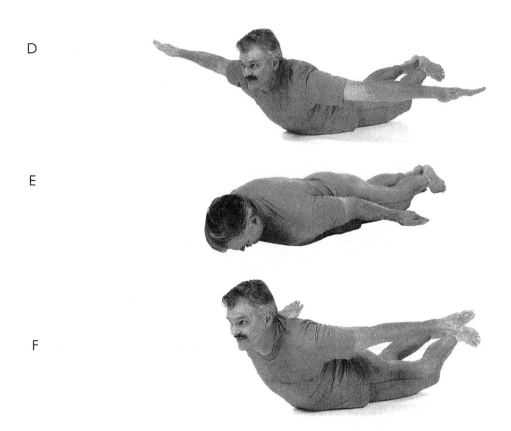

E

F

count of three as you lift in this position (D); breathe out to a count of three as you relax, and swing your arms back against your sides (E). Relax completely in this position. Now breathe in to a count of three as you lift (F); breathe out to a count of three as you relax, clasping your hands behind your back (G). Relax completely. Breathe in to a count of three as you lift again, straightening your arms as much as possible and lifting them away from your back (H). Breathe out to a count of three as you relax, bending your knees and holding on to your toes, feet, or ankles (I). Relax completely. Now breathe in to a count of three as you lift up for the fifth in the series, the Bow Pose (J), then breathe out

to a count of three as you relax, arms to your sides. Rest for several seconds, until your breath returns to normal and your body is completely relaxed.

When you have practiced these five positions for several days, you can add repetitions by reversing direction. When you reach the Bow Pose (position J), do it twice, then relax into the hands-clasped position, then lift and relax with arms at your sides, and so on back to the beginning Boat Pose with arms out in front. Repetitions: 1 to 5 sequences.

Keep your arms and legs straight.
Breathe in and hold breath in as you lift.
Relax completely between each two lifts.

G

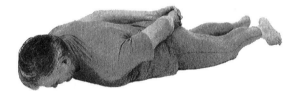

H

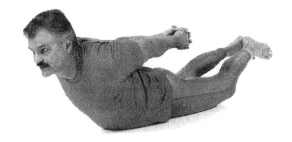

I

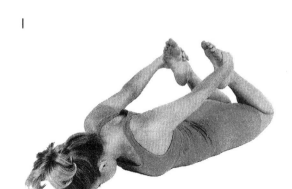

J

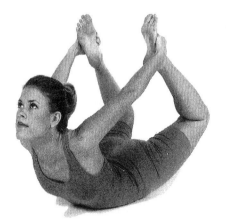

Easy Cobra Pose (Course 1)

- Limbers and straightens spinal column and back muscles
- Strengthens upper back and shoulders
- Prepares for Cobra Pose

Lie on your stomach, propped up on your elbows with hands clasped in front of you. Relax your head and shoulders so your head rests on or close to your hands (A). Breathe out to a count of three, then breathe in to a count of three as you lift your head, looking straight up at the ceiling. Hold for a count of three as you stretch up and back a little, stretching and compressing your spine without coming off your elbows (B). Be sure to relax your lower back so that you are curling rather than pushing up. Then relax and breathe out to a count of three as you lower your head back to your hands. Repetitions: 3.

Keep your elbows on the floor.
Relax your lower back.

A
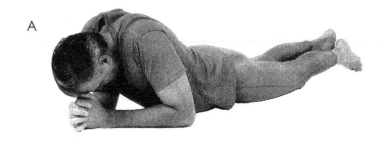

B
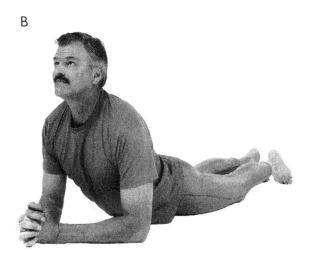

Cobra Pose (Courses 1, 2, & 3) (Bhujangasan)

- Improves function of intestines
- Increases body heat
- Strengthens back muscles and limbers spinal column
- Stimulates reproductive organs
- Increases overall body strength
- Strengthens eyesight
- Helps relieve impotence

Lie on your stomach with feet together, forehead on the floor, and palms flat on the floor under your shoulders (A). Your elbows will be up. Breathe in to a count of three as you raise your head—gaze up— then your chest, and finally your stomach, curling your spine rather than pushing with your arms (B). Be sure not to lift so high that your hipbones come off the floor. Try to use your back muscles to lift and your arms for balance and support only. Do not lift high enough to straighten your arms. Keep your lips together, and jut your lower jaw forward slightly to stretch the throat muscles. Hold the position for a count of three, then breathe out to a count of three as you uncurl slowly, keeping your head back until the very last. Your stomach touches first, then your chest, and finally your head, as you tuck your chin to chest and your forehead comes to rest on the floor. Relax until your breath returns to normal. This is a powerful exercise that brings energy to all parts of the body and balances the physical and emotional-spiritual bodies. Repetitions: 3.

Curl your spine using your back muscles
  rather than by pushing with your arms.
Your head should come up first and down last.
Hipbones must stay on the floor.

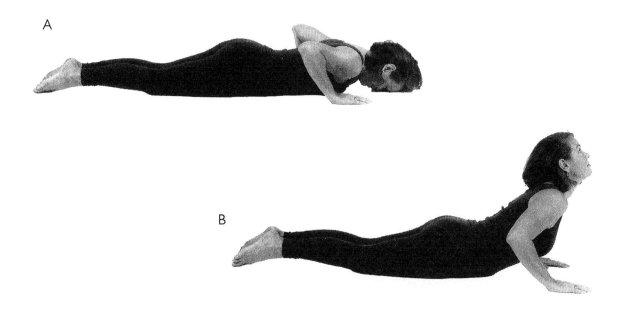

A

B

Bow Pose (Courses 1 & 2)
(*Dhanurasan*)

- Helps relieve chronic constipation
- Improves function of liver, kidneys, spleen, stomach, and intestines
- Strengthens back and thighs
- Aligns vertebrae properly
- Increases vigor and vitality
- Helps relieve impotence

Lie flat on your stomach with your forehead on the floor and bend your legs at the knees. Reach back and grasp both feet or ankles (A). Now breathe in to a count of three as you raise yourself, pulling your feet up and away from your body for a maximum stretch to the spine (B). Look up, and keep your lips together. Hold for a count of three, then breathe out to a count of three as you lower yourself to the floor. Repetitions: 3

Keep your eyes open, looking up.
Lift your feet up and away from your body.
Hold breath in as you lift.

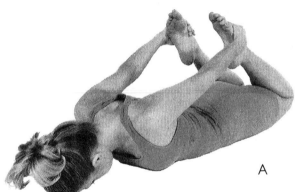

A

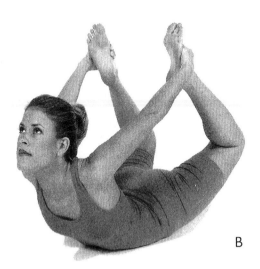

B

Sun Salutation (Courses 2 & 3)
(Surya Namaskar)

- Stimulates circulation throughout body
- Strengthens breathing muscles
- Limbers spine in both directions
- Stretches and strengthens hip and thigh muscles

Start in a standing position with palms together and close to your chest in the traditional greeting of India: Namaste (A). Breathe in to a count of three as you raise your arms in a wide circle overhead (B). Picture your arms bringing the sun up with the movement. At the top of the circle, touch your palms, stretch, and look up at your hands (C), holding your breath in for a count of three. Then breathe out to a count of three as you bend from the hips, keeping your head between your arms (D). Bend as far forward as possible, grasp your ankles, and pull your upper body toward your legs with your breath held out (E).

Now breathe in to a count of three as you lunge forward with your left foot (F). Raise your arms

A

B

C

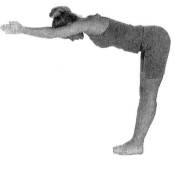

D

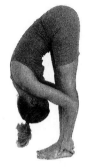

E

This is an important sequence that combines the stretching and strengthening functions of several major asans. Before trying this exercise, you should have begun the Course 2 routine and should be fairly proficient in the Standing Sun Pose, Cobra Pose, Thigh Stretch, and Cobra V-Raise. It is named the Sun Salutation because it is health-giving, like the sun. The sequence of movements represents the passage of the sun through the day and through the year.

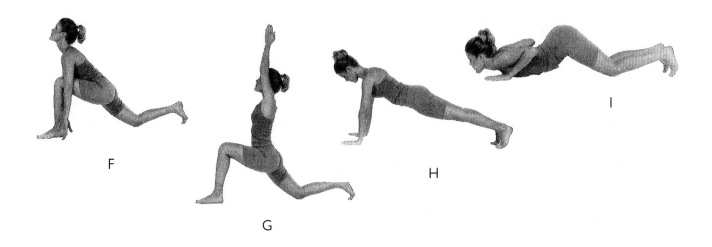

overhead, arching your back and pushing your hips forward to feel the stretch in your thighs (G). Look up and hold your breath in for a count of three. In the beginning keep your right knee on the floor. After a few weeks of practice, try holding the knee up.

Holding your breath in, lower your arms and bring your left leg back into a Plank Pose, arms straight and body on a plane (H).

Next, come down so that your knees, chest, hands, and chin are touching the floor in a zigzag position (I).

Breathe out to a count of three as you flatten your body, keeping your hands next to your shoulders (J).

Breathe in to a count of three as you arch up into a Cobra Pose (K).

Tuck your toes under and breathe out to a count of three, pushing your hips up into a V-Raise (L).

Breathe in to a count of three as you lunge forward with the right foot (M). Raise your arms in a wide circle overhead and look up (N). Hold for a count of three.

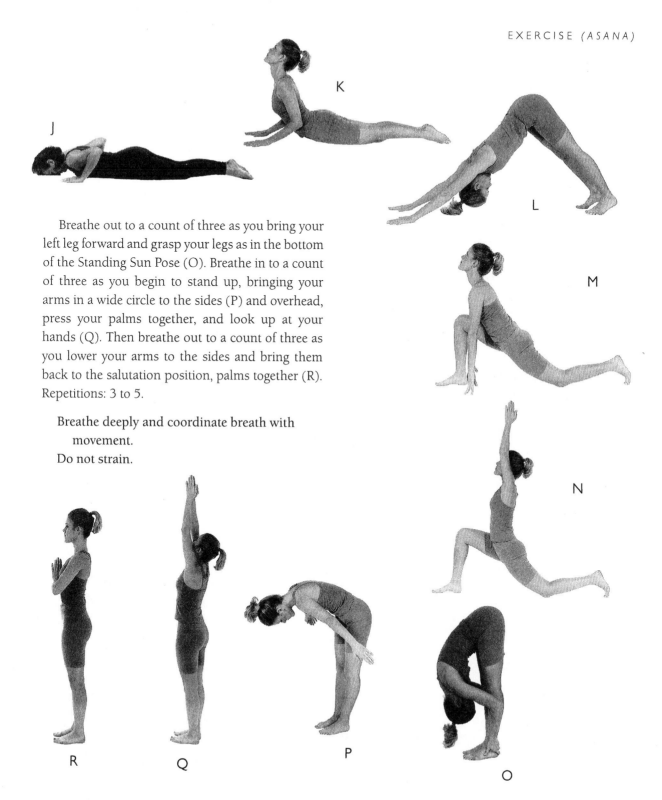

J

K

L

M

N

Breathe out to a count of three as you bring your left leg forward and grasp your legs as in the bottom of the Standing Sun Pose (O). Breathe in to a count of three as you begin to stand up, bringing your arms in a wide circle to the sides (P) and overhead, press your palms together, and look up at your hands (Q). Then breathe out to a count of three as you lower your arms to the sides and bring them back to the salutation position, palms together (R). Repetitions: 3 to 5.

Breathe deeply and coordinate breath with
    movement.
Do not strain.

R

Q

P

O

Chapter 5

ℬREATHING (PRANAYAMA)

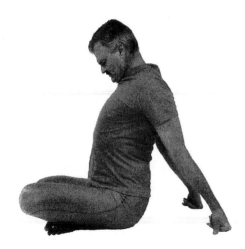

BREATHING TECHNIQUES

Breathing is probably the most important thing you do in life; in fact, without breath, you wouldn't be able to do anything at all! Breath is with you from the moment you are born until the instant you die. In between, your body usually automatically regulates how much air you breathe in and breathe out. Yet because it is so automatic, you probably do not think very much about your breath, unless you have been specifically trained in singing or sports or you have had illnesses that affected your respiration.

Yoga practice teaches that it is extremely beneficial to pay more attention to the breath, because the breath, body, and mind are so closely linked that a change in one immediately affects the other two. Consider what happens when, for example, you are at work and you receive a terse summons from the boss. As your mind goes through all the mistakes you might have made or the praise you hope to receive, your breath and body respond to your emotional state. Certain muscles become tense (notably those of the stomach, face, and shoulders); your breath becomes shallower and shorter; and other stress responses—such as increased pulse rate—are triggered. Another example: vigorous physical exercise can cause your breathing to become faster and deeper; after a certain point chemical changes in the body give the pleasurable experience of "runner's high."

In Yoga practice you learn how to take this concept one step further. By changing your breath pattern in specific ways, you can bring about beneficial changes in your body and mind. Remember a parent or teacher telling you, when you were upset, "Sit down and take a deep breath and you'll feel better"? In Yoga you learn how to do this systematically, so you experience consistent results. Yogic breathing techniques can be very effective tools for stress reduction.

My teacher Rama used to say that a person has one thought on inhalation and another on exhalation, so that the rate of breath determines the number of thoughts a person has. A greater number of thoughts (a faster breathing rate) thus results in less concentration, because there are so many thoughts going on:

As the number of ideas conceived by the mind increases, their power of fulfillment decreases; conversely, the fewer ideas the mind lingers over for a comparatively longer time, the greater their power of fulfillment, because these ideas are backed by the force of the mind. This force is called willpower. —Rama, "The World, a Fancy Tree" (quoted in Alice Christensen, Light of Yoga)

In your beginning Yoga practice, you learn how you can use correct breath patterns to enhance the effectiveness of your exercises (asans) and also to relax and quiet your mind in preparation for meditation. In this chapter you will learn the techniques you'll need for the breathing portion of your Yoga curriculum.

FACTS ABOUT YOGA AND YOUR BREATH

Oxygen is indispensable to proper metabolic function (defined as the physiological systems that provide energy to the body). Oxygen is used to break down—to oxidize—the protein, fats, and carbohydrates we eat for energy. Carbon dioxide and other waste products, along with a release of energy, are the end products of this process. The energy that is produced is what allows our muscles and other tissues to perform the work that we demand of them. Even the brain's tissues require oxygen for thinking, remembering, and other mental processes. In fact, the brain requires about three times as much oxygen as the rest of the body. Lack of oxygen nourishment can contribute to sluggishness, fatigue, confusion, loss of memory, and disorientation.

Yoga practice, especially asans and pranayamas, increases oxygen flow to the brain and body in several ways. It increases your vital capacity—the volume of air that you are able to forcibly exhale. Through Yoga practice the lung tissues may become more elastic, the joints of the ribs and spine become more supple, and the muscles that expand and contract the chest cavity become stronger.

Yoga asans stretch and strengthen postural muscles, contributing to an increase in tidal volume—the

Are you familiar with the sayings about getting up on the wrong side of the bed and starting off on the right foot? They are based on the notion that a person feels more balanced, more stable, when both sides of the nose are functioning approximately equally. When you first awake, you may notice that one side of your nose is more stopped up than the other. Before you stand up, notice which side is clear and put that foot down first, resting most of your weight for a few seconds on that side. For example, if your right side is stuffed up, put your weight down first on your left foot. The stuffed-up (right) side will clear up in a matter of minutes as you start moving around.

amount of air that flows in and out of the lungs in a normal resting state. As you read this, sit up straight and notice your breathing in its usual pattern. Now slouch down and see if you can notice how tidal volume is affected by poor posture.

A third way that Yoga practice ensures that the body and brain receive the oxygen they need is through improved blood circulation. The stretching of muscles that is accomplished through Yoga also means increased elasticity of the blood vessels, allowing improved blood flow—and thus more oxygen—to all parts of the body.

HOW TO START BREATHING BETTER

Try to breathe through your nose. Always try to inhale and exhale through your nose—never your mouth. This method is important in regulating the speed of your breath and improving your concentration. It helps to focus on the sound of your breath. If you close your throat slightly, you will hear a steamlike sound as you breathe in and out. Concentrating on this sound will help you keep your attention on your breath.

If one side of your nose is blocked, try this technique for opening it: If the right side is blocked, place your right fist in your left armpit. Drop your left arm and press in with your right fist. Hold for a few minutes until the right side of the nose opens. Reverse the procedure to open the left side. Another method is simply to lie on your side for a few minutes: if the right nostril is blocked, lie on your left side. Remember that although breathing through both nostrils equally is the ideal, you can still practice if your nose is partially blocked. The longer you practice Yoga, the more these passages will open.

Posture. Whether you sit cross-legged on the floor, sit on your feet, or sit on the edge of a chair, it is important to keep your back straight but relaxed, so that you don't ache and start slouching after a few minutes (A). If your hips and knees are limber enough to allow you to sit cross-legged on the floor, be sure to sit on one or more firm pillows to allow your hips to tilt forward. This lets your knees rest on the floor and makes a slight arch in your lower back (B). You may use any of the illustrated cross-legged

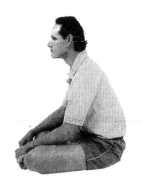

A

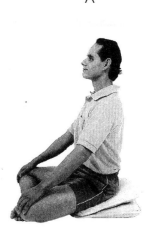

B

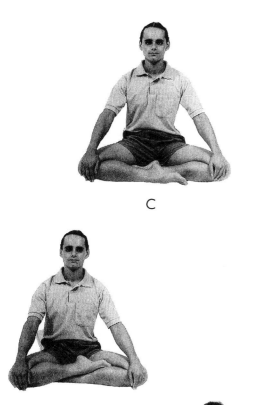

C

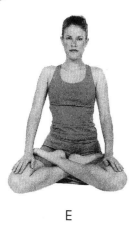

D

positions (C, D, E) that is comfortable. Do not try to force your legs into a painful position before they are ready; instead, do the hip- and knee-limbering asans every day in your routine until the joints in your hips, legs, and feet become more supple.

If you are sitting in a chair, sit on the edge—do not lean back. Tuck your toes under so your thighs are inclined forward slightly; if your feet don't reach the floor, put a pillow or book under them. If you are sitting on your feet, a small pillow under your ankles and another under your hips will be more comfortable (F). You can also straddle a firm pillow so that your legs are slightly separated (G).

Try each of these seated positions and see which feels most comfortable. Spend time on this now, and you will be rewarded by easier and more comfortable breathing practice.

E

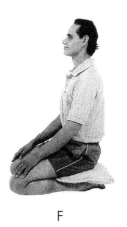

F

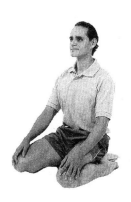

G

BREATH WARM-UPS

These exercises help loosen tight breathing muscles, relax your spine, and get your circulation going. If your feet or legs get cramped after doing these exercises, stop and move around, massage your feet and ankles, and then return to a comfortable seated position.

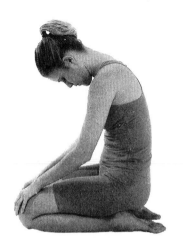

A

Back Arch

Slouch down so that your back is rounded as far forward as it will go, your chin is tucked into your chest, and your hands rest on your knees (A). Breathe in to a count of three as you arch your back forward, pushing your chest out and jutting your chin up (B). Keep lips together. Hold for a count of three, then breathe out to a count of three as you slouch again, remembering to tuck your chin. Repetitions: 3 to 5.

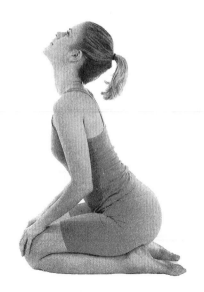

B

Arm Swing

Slouch forward as in the Back Arch, lifting straight arms in front of you until they are parallel to the floor (A). Breathe in to a count of three as you push your stomach and back forward into an arch while swinging your arms out to the sides and as far back as they will go. Keep them straight and parallel to the floor (B). Hold for a count of three, then breathe out to a count of three as you slouch, bringing your hands together in front. Repetitions: 3 to 5.

Variation: Bend your elbows and bring your arms back to the sides as if pulling back on the reins of a horse (C).

A

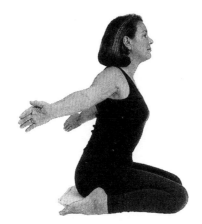

B

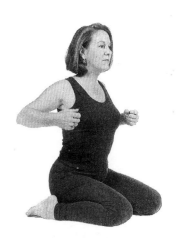

C

Arm Reach

Start with your arms at your sides (A). Breathe in to a count of three as you bring your arms out to the sides and up over your head in a wide circle. Stretch your arms directly up (B). Hold for a count of three, then breathe out and lower your arms to the sides again with the same circular motion. Repetitions: 3 to 5.

Variation: Make fists as you stretch your arms up.

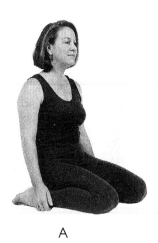

A

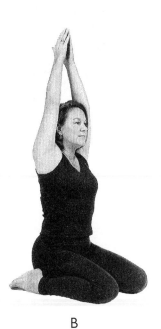

B

BREATHING EXERCISES (PRANAYAMAS)

Belly Breath

In a comfortable seated position, place your right hand on your abdomen, just below your navel, and the left against your lower back. Contract your abdominal muscles, then relax them. This is the main group of muscles you will be using in the Belly Breath. The purpose of doing the Belly Breath is to learn how to start breathing more deeply using your diaphragm first. You'll also learn how the breath can relax the stomach muscles when they are tensed because of stress.

First exhale and contract your belly muscles, pushing in with your right hand to reinforce the motion (A). Now relax your belly and inhale, pushing forward with your belly muscles—your right hand should be pushed forward, and there should be a slight arch in your lower back (B). Now exhale again, push in with your right hand, and flatten your back (do not slouch on the exhalation; just come back to a straight-back position). Repeat several times, trying to inhale and exhale as completely as possible each time. Tilt your pelvis forward to make a slight arch in the small of your back as you breathe in. Then return to a straight back as you tighten your stomach muscles and breathe out.

Do not hold your breath at any time, but try to make the breathing pattern smooth and steady. Breathe through your nose; you should feel the breath hitting the back of your throat first and hear a steamlike sound as the breath goes in and out. This sound is important, because achieving the proper sound helps you build greater control of the breath using your throat muscles.

In this exercise you will experience your diaphragm moving down to draw the air in and then up to expel the air. Most people breathe shallowly, with only the very top portion of the lungs. With the Belly Breath you draw more air down into the bottom portion of your lungs, increasing the oxygen absorbed into your bloodstream.

If you become light-headed during this exercise, stop and rest. As you continue daily practice, the light-headedness will disappear.

A

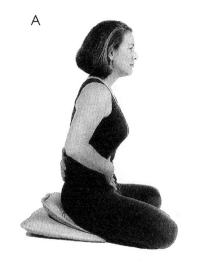

B

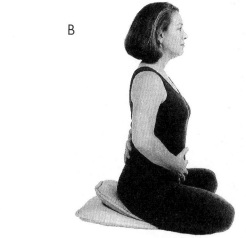

Complete Breath

The Complete Breath is a tool you can use anywhere, anytime, to calm your mind and relax. Using the Complete Breath to center yourself before your meditation and even before your asans will make those aspects of practice even more effective.

The Complete Breath has three major parts. You have already learned the first, by doing the Belly Breath. The second involves your rib cage. Place your hands on the lower part of your rib cage, with fingers just touching. As you breathe in, your rib cage expands—not just forward but also to the sides. When this happens, you will notice an increase in your breath capacity. As you inhale, remember to push the belly forward; there will be a slight arch in the lower back. Continue to breathe in and try to expand your ribs sideways (A); your fingers will naturally move apart. Do not strain. Exhale (B), and your fingers will come together again. Breathe steadily for several repetitions, keeping your hands on your ribs.

The third part of the Complete Breath concerns the top portion of the lungs. As you come to the top of your inhalation, straighten your shoulders, stretch your spine a little, and imagine the breath being pulled into the very top of your chest. Be careful not to strain.

Put the three stages together for the Complete Breath inhalation (C) and reverse for the exhalation (D). Inhalation is done from the bottom up and exhalation from the top down. Remember to breathe through your nose, concentrating on that steamlike sound in the back of your throat. Breathe evenly, without counting, and do not hold the breath at the top or bottom. Posture is important: your shoulders and head should stay essentially in the same position throughout. Try not to slouch forward on the exhalation.

Use the Wall Breath (E) to check your posture from time to time. Place a chair sideways against a wall and sit on it with your back against the wall. Be sure that your hips, shoulder blades, and back of

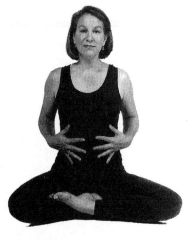

A

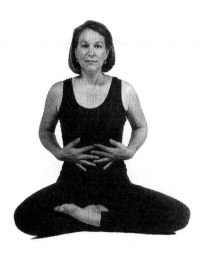

B

head are touching the wall. Start the Complete Breath with an exhalation, flattening the small of your back against the wall and tightening your stomach muscles. Now inhale and slightly arch your back as you fill up with air, using the three stages. Your shoulders and head should remain against the wall at all times. Repeat several times.

You can also practice this exercise lying on your back. As you breathe in, push your stomach up toward the ceiling. As you breathe out, tighten your stomach muscles and flatten the small of your back against the floor. Try this with a book on your stomach to strengthen your breathing muscles.

After a couple of weeks, start timing your breath, using a clock or watch with a second hand or a digital second readout. If you don't have either of these, simply count silently. Try to make your inhalation and exhalation about equal in length.

In the first ten weeks of the curriculum, try for an even, comfortable 10 seconds of inhalation and 10 seconds of exhalation. For most people the inhala-

tion is naturally shorter than the exhalation. Don't strain to extend the inhalation; instead, shorten your exhalation. Be sure not to hold your breath at either the top or the bottom, but make a smooth transition. Concentrate on the movement of your body and the sound of your breath. The evenness of the breath is more important than its length.

Practice the Complete Breath just before your meditation, to start the process of relaxation and help you become quiet internally.

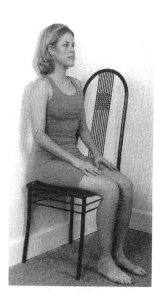

E

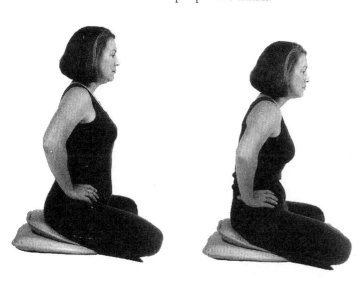

C   D

Earplugs

After you have practiced the Complete Breath for a few weeks, try it using earplugs. Your pharmacy probably has ear stopples made of wax, beeswax, or paraffin that are described as helpful for reducing environmental noise. (The rubber earplugs used for swimming are less effective.) Yogis have traditionally used earplugs to help them achieve greater smoothness and control over their breath.

Try closing your ears with your fingers and breathe deeply. Do you notice how much louder your breathing sounds, overriding any distracting sounds? This is the purpose of using earplugs. Knead them lightly to soften them, then flatten them on the outsides of your ear canals. Don't push them all the way in. Now practice the Complete Breath, trying to improve the evenness and smoothness of your breath.

You may find that this technique increases your concentration as well. If you wish, you can leave the earplugs in for meditation to reduce distracting noises.

Humming Breath

The Humming Breath departs from the pattern of breathing you have done so far, in which the inhalation and exhalation are of approximately equal length. In the Humming Breath the pattern is to breathe in for a short length of time and breathe out longer—as long as you can—while humming loudly and steadily. This exercise may seem strange at first, but it is extremely helpful in strengthening the diaphragm muscle and in quieting the mind for meditation.

Sitting comfortably, take in a full, quick Complete Breath (a little more quickly than you usually do—about 3 to 5 seconds), with the same movements of belly and chest. Now sing the word *hum* on one note and hold the *m* sound as you continue to exhale. Try to keep the tone steady and resonant until all your breath is gone. Then take in another deep, short Complete Breath and start again. Repetitions: at least 5.

Choose a pitch that is comfortable for your voice. In the beginning you may notice that the pitch wavers quite a bit; that is because you are learning to control your diaphragm all the way through the exhalation. Try not to let the sound die down at the end. You will have to push a little harder to keep a steady, resonant tone until the air has been completely exhaled.

BREATHING AND MOOD CHANGES

Earlier in this chapter we mentioned the ability of breathing exercises to change mood. Some exercises are especially useful for this purpose.

States of mind such as depression, upset, anger, and sadness can create a vicious cycle of tense muscles, negative thoughts, and constricted breathing. The following techniques are guaranteed to break that cycle and allow a more positive outlook to emerge.

Lion

Sit on your feet (or the edge of a chair) with your hands on your knees (A). Take in a deep complete breath, then exhale with a growl, opening your eyes, mouth, and hands wide, sticking out your tongue, and leaning forward (B). Repeat several times. Try this with a mirror. Look fierce.

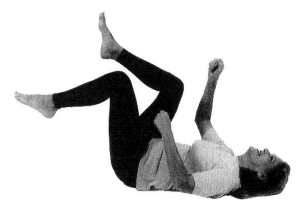

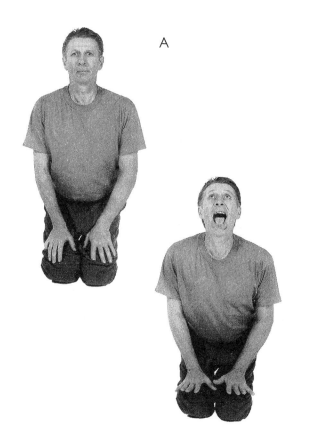

A

B

Laughasan

This exercise can be done sitting in a chair, but it is most effective when you can move your whole body, so I suggest you practice it lying down. Start your legs pumping in circles as if you were riding a bicycle. Pump your arms in circles as well, make fists, and laugh loudly. Get your whole body involved. Even if you have to start by pretending to laugh, you will end up really laughing, chasing your blues away.

BREATHING EXERCISES NEW TO COURSE TWO

Neti

Neti is a cleansing technique for the sinus passages. It helps clear those areas to facilitate breathing, and it can also be helpful in shrinking swollen membranes. Are you aware of the fact that modern medicine recommends lots of sweet or salty liquids when you have a cold and sore throat? The reason is that these types of liquids have what is called osmotic action, meaning that they draw liquid out of mucous membranes and help shrink swelling, thereby easing discomfort. Neti acts in much the same way.

Note: If you have allergies or a chronic sinus condition, do this technique only when the membranes are not inflamed.

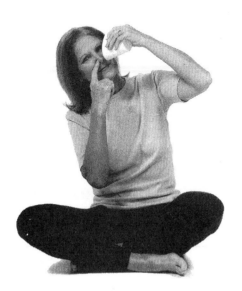

You will need a small Styrofoam or paper cup and table salt. Put about ½ teaspoon of salt in the cup and fill about halfway with warm (not cold) water. Stir.

Now press the sides of the cup together slightly so that you create a spout. Holding one nostril closed with a free finger, tip the cup toward your nose with your head tilted a little to the side with the closed nostril. Inhale and tip the cup at the same time, sniffing up a small amount of salt water into your nose. Tilt your head back so the water runs through your nasal passages. Soon you will feel it tickle the back of your throat. Try not to swallow. Instead, lean over a basin and spit out the water. Repetitions: 1 to 3 times each side. Gently wipe your nose, but don't blow hard for about 5 minutes.

It is not possible to drown from this technique! Practice it on a daily basis for a while and see if it makes your breathing more effective.

Kapalabhati

Kapalabhati is an important breath technique because it helps prepare the mind for meditation. The word *kapalabhati* means "shining skull." This breathing exercise helps to improve the nervous system coordination of the breath musculature, relieve stress by releasing muscle tension in the chest and belly muscles, and strengthen the diaphragm. Do not practice this technique when ill, during menstruation, or if you are taking tranquilizers.

It is mandatory that your back be straight and your pelvis tilted forward so there is a slight arch in the small of your back and your knees touch the floor. Put a pillow under your hips to help attain the correct posture. If you cannot sit comfortably on the floor, practice this technique sitting on the edge of a chair. Your hips must be higher than your knees. This is important because you won't be able to get the proper movement if you are using your lower back or stomach muscles to maintain a comfortable sitting position.

Here is the beginning sequence, followed by an explanation of each item:

One-half normal breath inhalation, then

1. 10 seconds Bellows Breath (approximately 1 per second)
2. Complete, quick exhalation (3 to 5 seconds)
3. Complete, quick inhalation (3 to 5 seconds)
4. Hold breath in for 2 to 3 seconds
5. Exhale as long as possible
6. 5 or more regular breaths, until breath is back to normal

1. BELLOWS BREATH

As its name implies, the Bellows Breath is a rapid in-and-out movement of the diaphragm. Place your hands just below your ribs in the center of your torso. For the Bellows Breath, you will be taking much smaller and faster breaths than normal, but move enough air so that you hear the steamlike sound in the back of your throat.

Notes on speed and intensity: For the first week concentrate on evenness in speed and intensity in this breath. Do not emphasize the inhalation or the exhalation. The best way to ensure this is to start slowly: one in-and-out cycle each second for 10 seconds. Try to make it a concentrated but very controlled burst of air both in and out, so that you are inhaling and exhaling the same amount of air. After a few weeks, if you are maintaining a smooth, even, and steady bellows, increase the speed to two in-and-out breaths per second. After several weeks you can try increasing to three per second, but do not go faster than that.

Do you notice any light-headedness after doing the bellows? If so, you may be using the top part of your chest rather than your belly and diaphragm. Check by placing your hands on your chest. If you feel excessive movement, try to relocate the movement downward. Heavy smokers may experience dizziness even if they are breathing correctly; if so, reduce the number of bellows you do at one time to five—or even fewer.

2. QUICK EXHALATION

Use the same complete exhalation procedure as for the Complete Breath, only faster (3 to 5 seconds). Don't slouch. Use your stomach muscles. Get all the air out.

3. QUICK INHALATION

Use the same inhalation procedure as in the Complete Breath, only faster (3 to 5 seconds). Fill from the bottom. Fill completely. Check your posture.

4. HOLD BREATH

This short (2 to 3 seconds) hold is to center or focus your awareness fully on the moment of stillness that is the transition between the inhalation and the exhalation.

5. EXHALE AS LONG AS POSSIBLE

This segment of the breath allows you to enter the most absorbing and focused part of this exercise. The idea is to extend your exhalation as long as possible without strain. Imagine the breath coming out in the thinnest, softest stream you can imagine. Close your eyes to increase your concentration. Try to focus only on the sound of your breath (in the back of the throat). Be sure not to strain to the point of "squeaking" as you exhale. Also, don't extend the breath so much that you are starved for breath when finished. Stretch your exhalation a few seconds further each week. In the beginning your exhalation will be about 15 to 20 seconds. By the time you have completed the Course 2 ten-week session, if you've practiced regularly, your exhalation may have grown to 30 seconds or more.

6. 5 OR MORE REGULAR BREATHS

Release your breath and let it come naturally until the rate is back to normal and your muscles have relaxed (five or more breaths).

REPETITIONS

Repeat the whole sequence 3 times to begin. If that feels comfortable and you have extra time, you can increase to 5 repetitions after a few weeks.

Suggested Kapalabhati rate sequence during Course 2

Weeks 1 and 2: Bellows 10 seconds; whole sequence 3 times

Weeks 3 and 4: Bellows 20 seconds; whole sequence 3 times

Weeks 5 and 6: Bellows 20 seconds but increase speed to 2 per second; whole sequence 3 times

Weeks 7 and 8: Bellows 30 seconds; whole sequence 5 times

Weeks 9 and 10: Bellows 30 seconds; increase speed to 3 per second if ready; whole sequence 5 times

Bramari Breath

The Bramari Breath is a focusing exercise that demands attention, much like the Humming Breath, because you have to make an audible sound. In this case it is an extended *zzz* sound, hence its name, which means "bee breath."

Start by placing your fingers horizontally across your face (A): thumbs on the flaps in front of the ears; first fingers on the lashes of your closed eyes; second fingers at the nostrils; third and fourth fingers at the corners of the mouth. Fingers should be placed lightly, not pressing hard. By symbolically closing your sensory organs, you reinforce the idea of focusing on the sound of the breath alone. Do not apply pressure, except with your thumbs, which should gently close the ear openings on the exhalation so that the sound is intensified.

Inhale completely through your nose, using all three steps as in the Complete Breath. As you exhale, press your thumbs softly to close the ears and

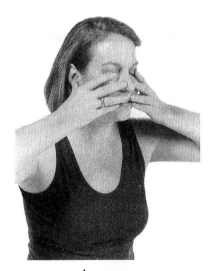

A

make the *zzz* sound, extending the breath and keeping the tone steady until you run out of air. Repetitions: 3 to 5.

Most students find this an excellent technique for changing moods, because it forces concentration away from the uncomfortable mood—very much like a radio station that doesn't stay on its frequency—and clears the mind. Its focusing effects help quiet the mind for meditation.

BREATHING EXERCISES NEW TO COURSE THREE

Spinal Arch

The Spinal Arch stimulates the nerves of the entire spinal column and places pressure on the rib cage and lungs, allowing more oxygen to be absorbed through the lung walls. It is part of the Emotional Stability Routine (Course 3).

Sit cross-legged, and place your fists on the floor directly behind your hips (A). Take a partial breath in (to about one-half normal capacity), straighten your arms so that you are lifting a little of your weight off your buttocks, arch your back slightly, tuck your chin to your chest, and contract your rectal muscles (B). This contraction is called the Mulabhanda lock. Hold your breath and the pose for 3 to 6 seconds. Release and relax. Repetitions: 3.

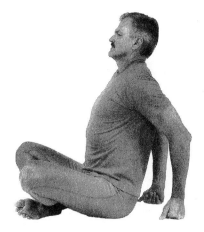

A

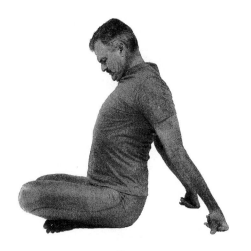

B

Agni Kriya

This is an advanced breath exercise that should be attempted only after you have become proficient in Kapalabhati. Agni Kriya involves what is called a *bandha,* or lock, of a part of the body, in order to intensify a movement or limitation of movement of energy. In Agni Kriya you have to practice isolating your stomach and diaphragm muscles. This is a powerful technique that should never be done on a full stomach, by pregnant women, or during the menstrual period.

First practice this exercise from a standing posi-tion. Place your hands on your bent knees, fingers pointed in (A), bracing yourself but relaxed. Breathe in deeply, filling your lungs as fully as possible; then breathe out very quickly, through pursed lips. Did you get all the air out? Try to exhale a little more. Now hold your breath out and pull in and up with your stomach muscles, contracting them so that the triangular area under your rib cage becomes slightly hollow (B). Tuck your chin toward your chest. Hold for a moment. Now release your muscles and lift your chin a little. When your muscles are com-pletely relaxed, release and breathe in. Relax until

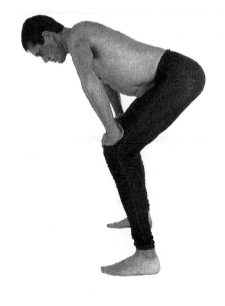

A

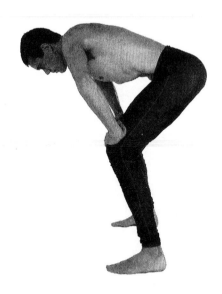

B

your breath returns to normal (take five or more normal, resting breaths).

Practice 3 repetitions of this first step after your other breath exercises every day. If you experience headaches, nervousness, pain in the diaphragm, or dizziness, stop the exercise; your nervous system is not yet strong enough to support it. Continue with daily asans, Complete Breath, and Kapalabhati, and try again in a few weeks.

If you experience none of these symptoms after a week, begin repetitions of the stomach contraction as follows: Exhale completely through pursed lips, hold the breath out, draw the stomach up and in, hold for a moment, then release the stomach muscles but not the held breath. Contract the stomach again; release; contract a third time; release. Relax the stomach muscles completely, then breathe in and relax until your breath returns to normal (five or more normal, resting breaths). This is one repetition. Repetitions: 3.

After practicing this exercise standing for a while, try it seated (C and D). To ensure that your hips are higher than your knees, use a pillow or two or sit on your feet. You can also do this seated on the edge of a sturdy chair.

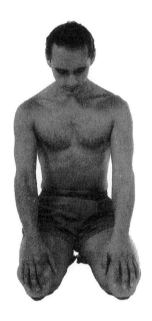

C

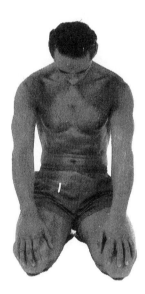

D

Chapter 6

ℛELAXATION AND MEDITATION

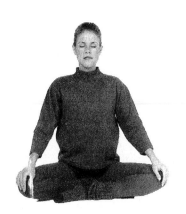

Meditation is an opportunity for new experience—something you have never seen or known before. It opens the door for direct communication between your outer physical and your inner emotional-spiritual bodies. Because each person's meditation experience is slightly different, it is important not to compare your experiences with those of other students—or even to compare one day's experience with that of another. Do not judge your experience as good or bad. This is a mistake. Meditation cannot be judged; simply "put in your time." The best way to approach meditation is to make a daily commitment to it. Practice becoming still; then watch what happens.

Meditation cannot be forced. If you take a competitive, forceful attitude toward attaining stillness, you will probably have more difficulty than if you simply let go and relax into it.

If you are in a class, your teacher may use a relaxation procedure similar to what is described here. To get the most out of your daily practice session, go through the relaxation sequence just as you remember it from class. You can also read the instructions slowly into a tape recorder and play the tape back while you relax. A prerecorded audiocassette of relaxation and meditation is available from the American Yoga Association (see Resources).

If you are using this book as your teacher, take some time to familiarize yourself with the relaxation process by reading this section through carefully and visualizing each part of your body in sequence. Then get into position, close your eyes, and try to approximate the sequence as best you can remember. Start at your forehead, move down your body to your toes, and then come back up your spine to the top of your head. Do not worry if you forget one or two points, but be sure to spend adequate time (at least 4 minutes) on relaxation before moving on to your meditation.

It is important to take the time to relax completely, because relaxation will begin the process of internalization. Use your Yoga mat or blanket, and wear your exercise clothes. Put on a pair of socks, and wrap a blanket or shawl around yourself. Do not meditate in a draft. Turn your telephone off and put a sign on your door so that you will not be disturbed. Make sure pets are in another room so that they will not disturb you. If you are practicing meditation at the end of the day, it is a good idea to bathe first, to relax and imagine the removal of stressful associations that have accumulated during the day. You will find other hints for getting more out of your meditation practice after the description of the process itself.

HOW TO BEGIN

1. Get into Position

Start your meditation practice by lying on your back on your mat or blanket. (See Chapter 10 for a shorter seated meditation procedure that you can use at any time of day.) If your blanket is shorter than you are, make sure your head rests on it. Are you warm enough? Turn off any overhead lights so they don't glare into your eyes. Close your eyes. Do not use a pillow under your head unless, because of injury or your doctor's orders, you must keep your head elevated. Let your arms relax at your sides, with the palms facing up. Let your legs and feet relax. Check to make sure that your body is very straight. This position is called the Corpse Pose (*Shavasan*) because the body gets so completely relaxed that it is almost motionless—only a slight breathing motion is apparent (A). If your lower back feels tense or strained, you may place a pillow or two under your knees.

In beginning classes we start with the Corpse Pose because in it the mind can be completely free from worry about the body—there is no discomfort from the back or legs to intrude upon the experience. In the second ten-week class we begin to experiment with seated meditation. There are many variations to a seated position (see p. 144), but the important thing to remember—just as in postures for breathing—is that there should be a slight arch in the back to prevent slouching and strain. Use the same pillows you use for your breathing exercises (B).

If you meditate immediately after your breathing exercises, you may want to stretch your legs and massage your knees and ankles before going on to

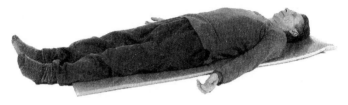

A

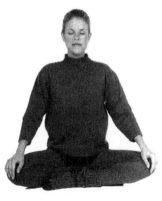

B

meditation. Don't hold a sitting position to the point of pain or numbness. When discomfort starts to distract you from your meditation, gently shift to the Corpse Pose without opening your eyes and with as little movement as possible. Then quickly go through the relaxation process that follows, checking to make sure that the special tension trouble areas, such as the breath, face, and stomach, are relaxed, and continue your meditation.

2. Relax Completely

Spend 4 to 6 minutes going through the steps in this process. When your body is relaxed and still, it will be much easier to quiet your mind. Do not worry if you cannot recall the entire procedure; just remember to move your attention slowly from your forehead down to your toes and back up your spine to your head, relaxing each part individually.

First, mentally detach yourself from all the activities, responsibilities, and cares that occupy you during the day. Say to yourself, "For a few minutes I don't have to speak, move, or respond to anyone or anything. I don't even have to think. I can become completely still and relaxed."

FACE

To begin your relaxation, bring your concentration or attention to the area of your forehead between the eyebrows and quietly imagine a diamondlike dot of light. This is the part of the body that represents a stage of consciousness called the Ajna Chakra. If you can't imagine this light, or if trying to do so makes you uncomfortable, just concentrate your attention on the area between your eyebrows.

Now take your attention down your nose bone and across your eyebrows, relaxing them. Let the force of gravity and your attention relax all the muscles in the forehead and eyes. The eyes merit special attention because they are the center for perception, the primary sense organs through which we perceive and respond to the world. Allow your eyes to sink back into their sockets until the muscles and nerves feel relaxed and completely stilled.

Move your attention across your cheeks, relaxing the muscles underneath your skin. Focus for a few seconds on the hinges of your jaws, located just in front of your ears. Relax your jaws as much as possible. You can even let your mouth hang open slightly to relax your lower jaw as much as possible. Relax your mouth, and picture your teeth, tongue, and throat.

Remind yourself that you don't have to speak for a few minutes. Now move your attention to your neck and throat. Imagine that your face and throat are made out of warm, soft wax. Relax your neck and throat.

SHOULDERS, ARMS, HANDS

Move your attention across your collarbone, relaxing it, and then move to your shoulders. Pause for a moment and picture your shoulder joints loosening and relaxing. Direct your attention down your arms.

Picture the long bones in your arms, the skin, muscles, nerves, and veins in your elbows all becoming still and relaxed. Imagine your wrists and hands floating in water. Don't move your hands; just relax them from the inside with your mind. Visualize the position of your hands, the shapes of your fingers and nails, the lines in your hands, and then let them go limp, just as a baby's hands curl when it is asleep.

HEART AND LUNGS

Gently redirect your attention to your chest. Picture your heart pumping steadily. Then take a deep breath, and as you exhale imagine your heart relaxing even more than it already has. It doesn't have to beat quite as hard now for a few minutes. Rest your heart.

BREATH

Observe how your breathing pattern is becoming more and more relaxed. Take another deep breath. As you fill your lungs, picture them as bright, strong, and healthy, and exhale in a long sigh, letting your lungs relax back into your natural breath pattern. Don't try to slow or speed up your breath; let it become smooth, quiet, and rhythmic, free from all tension or strain.

STOMACH AND INTERNAL ORGANS

Even if you aren't quite sure what they look like, picture your internal organs—your stomach, liver, kidneys, intestines, and so on, and relax them. Imagine them working perfectly. Imagine your insides gently sinking toward your backbone.

HIPS, LEGS, FEET

Let the bones, muscles, glands, and nerves in your pelvis and hip joints all become still and free from strain or tension. Continue down your legs, picturing the long muscles, nerves, and bones sinking limply toward the floor, like warm putty. Relax the joints of the knees, picturing the veins as you relax them. Relax your ankles, feet, and toes, and picture your toes. Think of their shape and the position of your feet. Let your feet become limp and relaxed. Relax your heels where they touch the floor, and imagine that the floor is relaxed where your heels touch it.

SPINAL COLUMN

Gently bring your attention to the base of your spine. Picture your spinal column as a gently curving elevator with the spinal cord running up inside it like a shiny line of electricity to the brain. Relax your spinal column nerves and bones from your lower back up to the back of your neck. Then relax the spot where your spinal column joins your skull. Release any tension from the back of your neck. Picture the brain, and let it become absolutely relaxed. Feel as though it is relaxing and settling quietly into your skull.

RECHECK FACE

Check your face for any lingering tension, especially in the area of your eyes. Drop your lower jaw and relax it. Now gently bring your attention back to the space in the forehead between the eyebrows. Your whole body is now quiet and relaxed.

3. Think of the Sound Om

Start your meditation period by thinking of the sound *Om* (pronounced "ohm"). This word is a mantram, a sound formula that has a specific effect on the mind when it is repeated or heard. *Om* is the oldest and most basic sound in classical Yoga. It has been said that if you could hear the subtle humming sound of the collective atomic structure of your own body and mind, that sound would most resemble *Om*.

Classical Yoga uses the sound *Om* to center and focus the mind. Try to empty your mind except for the sound itself, which will eventually lead to complete silence. When you meditate, try repeating the sound mentally a few times after you complete your relaxation. You may find that this helps you to become quiet.

4. Be Quiet and Still for 10 to 20 Minutes

As your attention starts to shift from your relaxed body to your mind, begin to observe and detach yourself from involvement with your thoughts. Meditation is a state of complete stillness and inactivity within the conscious mind. There may still be thoughts and perceptions moving at the edges of your awareness, but your attention is nevertheless focused on the silence and stillness that surround and underlie thought. Try to stop thinking. Stop all thought. Think nothing.

5. Helpful Hints

Meditation is not the same as being unconscious. In meditation, your body is completely relaxed, just as it is in sleep, but your mind is attentive, alert, and poised. Try to adopt an attitude of playfulness instead of a forceful one of pushing or pressing against your thoughts. Remember that you are attempting to experience stillness—something that, for most people, may be a completely new experience. Like any other type of training, meditation takes practice.

At first you will become aware of stillness after the fact, when you start thinking and realize that you had not been thinking for a few seconds previously. If you catch yourself in the middle of a thought, finish it, but then consciously let it fade away and try to focus on the silence in the mind before the next thought arises. Try to experience the characteristics of the silence—its wideness, deepness, thickness, texture, and so on.

Even if you feel that you are still for only a few seconds at a time at first, those periods will gradually lengthen and widen. The experience of stillness will become engrossing and pleasant.

Sometimes you may fall asleep. If this happens, just remember that as you begin to meditate you are giving your body all the cues it associates with sleep—a darkened room, relaxing the body, lying down, closing your eyes—so it is natural for you to slip into this state sometimes, especially if you are very fatigued. If this happens to you, you may experience a kind of sleep different than usual: probably deeper and more restful, and usually without dreams. You may also notice that you tend to wake up spontaneously after 20 or 30 minutes feeling refreshed. As you continue to practice, the sleep state will pass.

Try not to set an alarm when you meditate, because the loud sound will jar your nervous system and startle you awake too violently. If you meditate in the morning and are afraid you will fall asleep and be late for work, you may wish to consider sitting up for your meditation (see p. 144 for seated positions). When you meditate, tell your mind to inform you of the time you wish to end your meditation. It will do that.

Sometimes, there may be so many thoughts going through your mind that it becomes very hard to be still. On those days you can try using an image of some kind to help relax your mind. Pick an image that gives you a quiet feeling, such as a lake, ocean, meadow, sky, or the like, and visualize that image until you experience the same kind of quiet feeling. Then gently let go of the image—just let it dissolve—and stop thinking.

In Chapter 5 you read about using earplugs to increase your concentration on the sound of your breath. If you wish, you can also use the earplugs during meditation. In the beginning stages of meditation practice, external sounds, such as a clock, traffic, or air conditioner, may seem to become much louder. This is because your internal thoughts are no longer masking them. After a while these sounds will not bother you.

6. Coming Out of Meditation

When your meditation period is over, repeat the sound *Om*. Then, before you move, try to remember how it feels to be still inside. You can remember that feeling whenever you wish during the day, and it will remain with you.

Never jump right up after your meditation. Move slowly. Start by changing your breathing pattern. Breathe a little more deeply, and picture the air filling and waking your body. Wiggle your fingers and make fists. Wiggle your toes. Pull your toes back toward your face so you feel a stretch up the backs of your legs. Whenever you are ready, stretch like a cat and slowly begin to move about.

BENEFITS OF MEDITATION IN EVERYDAY LIFE

If you practice meditation every day, even for just a few minutes, you will soon notice that the rest and relaxation you feel during practice will begin to suffuse your entire life. These periods of stillness can be as refreshing as an hour's nap, because for a few minutes you are taking a mental vacation from all the cares, responsibilities, upsets, concerns, and conversations of your daily life. The practice of Yoga meditation opens you to the voice and experience of your inner body. Through Yoga, you can become a truly whole person with a balanced outlook from both your physical and emotional-spiritual bodies.

The mind changes its shape through perception, imagination, desire, emotion, daydreaming, reasoning, and many other mental processes. These are like waves or ripples on the surface of a pond, which obscure the view of the bottom. Yoga teaches the mind to assume the shape of whatever thought occupies it, just as water takes on the shape of whatever container it is in. Meditation teaches your mind to take the shape of silence. Meditation is the quieting of those mental thought waves so that your inner body can make itself known. You feel complete. You realize that true happiness does not come from other people or from going places, buying things, eating and drinking, or taking drugs. Happiness comes from within you.

COMMON EXPERIENCES IN MEDITATION

Part of Your Body—or All of It— Seems to Disappear

When you completely relax in meditation, the senses—including the kinesthetic sense, which is the awareness of where your body is in space—withdraw into the inner emotional-spiritual body.

You Feel Light or Heavy

When your awareness begins to shift from physical consciousness to the inner emotional-spiritual body, you'll sometimes feel lightness or heaviness. This experience is similar to the feeling of falling when going to sleep that sometimes jerks your body awake.

You See Lights or Colors, or Hear Sounds

Seeing lights or colors or hearing sounds during meditation is often a very seductive experience, caused by becoming more aware of the electrical activity in the brain, which then manifests as light or sound. You may read about the meanings of different colors and images, but we encourage students simply to note—and later record, if you're so inclined—these experiences, and go on toward the experience of stillness.

A Solution to a Problem Suddenly Occurs to You

If you have ever gone to sleep with a problem unsolved and woken up with the answer, you will understand how meditation helps encourage the intuitive voice of the inner body. When you quiet the physical body, you are welcoming the inner emotional-spiritual body, whose voice is intuition and creativity. Although it's best not to think of your meditation primarily as a problem-solving session, you might consider keeping a pad of paper and a pen close at hand so that if something important occurs to you, you can write it down, then continue with your meditation in stillness, instead of ending your meditation early or being anxious about holding on to the insight.

You Feel Cold

Your body temperature naturally drops a bit as you relax, so be prepared by wearing socks and wrapping your torso in a sweater or blanket before you begin.

Your Eyes Twitch

The eye muscles are usually the last muscle group in your body to relax. You may notice a correlation between periods of thought and movement of your eyes—similar to the rapid eye movement (REM) that occurs as you dream. As your ability to quiet internal conversation improves, your eye muscles will gradually relax. If the difficulty persists, it may be wise to check your diet; a B vitamin deficiency may be indicated.

Chapter 7

DIET AND NUTRITION

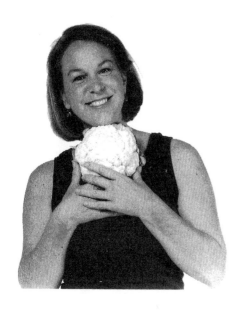

My interest in diet goes back to when my two-year-old son developed asthma. As I was searching for help, I came across the just-published book *Let's Get Well* by Adelle Davis. I had the good fortune to talk with her personally, and she offered a host of valuable and effective nutritional advice that helped my son tremendously. He eventually grew to 6 feet, 8 inches, and played two varsity sports in high school. Through this experience Adelle and I became friends. Several years later she met Rama and me in Virginia Beach, where she and I were speaking on the same program. Adelle later helped me when I developed a coal tar allergy, with severe symptoms triggered by artificial food coloring and flavoring. She was also a great help in reducing the angina pain that Rama was experiencing at the time.

These experiences helped to convince me that the conventional nutritional wisdom—that the typical American diet met all our nutritional needs and that food additives were safe and beneficial—was suspect. Yoga entered my life about this same time, and educating myself about nutrition became part of my immersion in Yoga.

It is simple common sense for someone who is beginning Yoga practice to consider the strong effect diet has on one's body and mind. Our daily food choices and habits can affect our long-term health as well as our moment-to-moment state of mind. In this chapter I will talk about why it makes sense to follow a healthy diet from both physical and philosophical perspectives. I will also outline the American Yoga Association's approach to healthy eating, which includes a vegetarian diet.

Here are some of the health advantages of a really good diet:

- *Renewed vitality* for activities such as Yoga practice
- *Preventing/postponing chronic diseases* such as heart disease, high blood pressure, diabetes, some cancers, and arthritis
- *Achieving/maintaining ideal weight.* Recent studies have shown that the majority (54 percent) of American adults are overweight, and about 20 percent of these are clinically obese. Obesity and diabetes are rising at alarming rates in children as well. Although young children need a certain amount of essential fatty acids in their diets, most children eat too much saturated fat, mostly from junk foods.

Experts have known for years that most Americans eat too little of the right foods and too much of the wrong foods, and they generally agree on how to improve the situation. The Yoga philosophy of diet that I describe in this chapter lines up directly with the majority of these recommendations. Here are some general recommendations for the average healthy adult:

- Eat a wide variety of the right kinds of foods—whole grains, fruits and vegetables, reduced-fat dairy products, and protein from legumes. This is still the best way to ensure adequate nutrition. Avoid excessive intake of foods high in saturated fat, sugar, and salt.
- Maintain your ideal weight by eating fewer calories when you are less active. Preventing weight gain and obesity is much easier than losing excess weight and keeping it off. If you are overweight now, there's just one way to change that: by eating fewer fat calories and

fewer calories overall than you expend in activity. No matter what the popular diet books tell you, no other means really works over the long term. Most experts agree that vegetarians tend to weigh less, probably because they eat more foods high in complex carbohydrates, compared with the more calorie-dense, high-fat and high-protein meat, poultry, and fish.

- Add more whole-grain cereals and breads, and more fruits and vegetables to your diet. Not only are these foods the best sources of vitamins and minerals, but they also provide complex carbohydrates to sustain energy, and fiber to clean the intestines and keep cholesterol in check. More important, each serving is a cocktail of natural phytochemicals, which are loaded with health-enriching benefits. These nutritious foods will also help ensure a diet that is low in fat.
- Eat less total fat, particularly saturated fat (such as from meat and butter) and cholesterol. Also limit foods containing hydrogenated or partially hydrogenated fats, or those high in trans–fatty acids, such as commercial frying oil, pastries made with vegetable shortening, and most stick margarines. All these fat sources raise cholesterol levels. Some individuals are more susceptible to both saturated fat and cholesterol and their ability to raise blood fats, so it seems smart to err on the side of caution. Replace vegetable oil with extra-virgin olive, canola, or peanut oil (especially for high-temperature cooking such as stir-frying), because these monounsaturated fatty acids resist oxidation and help your arteries stay plaque-free. Boost your intake of essential omega-3 fatty acids with 1

teaspoon of flaxseed oil per day. Flaxseed oil is good for low-temperature cooking and uncooked uses such as salad dressings.

- Avoid eating refined carbohydrates in the form of sugar or white-flour products (soda, candy, sweet pastries, pies, cakes, and cookies) as much as possible. Did you know that a third of American adults get almost half of their daily calories from junk foods?
- Avoid eating too much heavily salted food or processed foods, which often contain large amounts of sodium.
- If you drink alcoholic beverages, do so in moderation. Most experts recommend that men should never exceed two drinks per day, and women one. One drink consists of 12 ounces of beer, 4 ounces of wine, or 1 ounce of liquor.

THE VEGETARIAN DIET AND HEALTH

Vegetarian diets have become very popular; the number of Americans who describe themselves as vegetarians has more than doubled in the past ten years. It is now estimated that one in ten Americans consider themselves vegetarians. That's not to say none of them ever eats meat. Recently 20 percent of vegetarians reported that they ate meat at least once a month and fish and poultry more often, leading some to describe this type of diet as "near vegetarian." Vegetarians may include dairy products such as milk, yogurt, and cheese in their diets (they are called lactovegetarians), as we recommend, and sometimes eggs. This is very close to the ideal diet as described in the classical texts of Yoga and by my teachers. Vegetarians who refuse all animal prod-

ucts, including eggs and dairy, are usually called vegans, some limiting their diet to fruit or raw foods.

Vegetarians have a greatly reduced death rate from all major causes, probably as a result of many factors. These include eating more fruits, vegetables, and polyunsaturated fatty acids, and less saturated fat, cholesterol, and alcohol than the rest of the population. Also, vegetarians tend to have a healthier lifestyle; generally they smoke less, weigh less, and are more physically active. Ongoing research is devoted to identifying the specific phytochemicals in fruits and vegetables that are responsible for vegetarians' overall better health.

WHY IS DIET IMPORTANT IN YOGA?

Yogis stress the importance of a moderate and disciplined diet for a number of reasons, the two major ones being ethical and psychological.

Diet and Ethics

Nonviolence is the foundation of all ethical observances and restraints (yamas and niyamas, see Chapter 11). Through Nonviolence comes a sense of connection to all forms of life. Perceiving all life as sacred is an outgrowth of the practice of Nonviolence, and most practitioners feel that using animals as a food source is an unnecessary act of violence. Many students experience a noticeable reduction in their own fear and anxiety when they begin to practice Nonviolence. The classic vegetarian diet of fruits, vegetables, grains, and dairy foods, prepared fresh, enhances this experience.

Many Americans today are choosing to eat less or no meat for ethical reasons. Raising animals and processing their meat is a relatively inefficient means of food production. The grains and legumes fed to animals could nourish many more people than the meat from the animals themselves. An ethical concern for the rights of animals also motivates many Americans. Livestock are commonly raised and slaughtered under dreadful conditions. Other Americans are understandably concerned about health issues, such as the growing biohazards created by mass food production, pollutants and bacteria introduced into meat products by substandard processing practices, and toxicity from heavy metals in many fish.

Diet and State of Mind

A primary tenet of Yoga philosophy is that the state of the body and breath directly affects the mind—this is the key reason for practicing asans, pranayamas, and the other techniques of Yoga.

Yoga techniques give extra attention to the physical body because the body affects the mind. It can enhance or hamper mental function. Yoga techniques are often misunderstood, especially in the West, as a form of physical culture, yet they are ultimately a path to the metaphysical. Asans and breath exercises are designed to promote health and a balanced nervous system so there is no impediment to advanced practices of concentration and meditation. Similarly, Yoga's ancient manuals also prescribe a fresh, whole-food, vegetarian diet to strengthen the mental effects of the techniques.

We have all experienced mental dullness, moments or longer periods when we just cannot seem to concentrate. You have probably also noticed times when your mind is so nervous you feel like a child with attention deficit disorder—too jittery to focus on one thing for more than a few seconds. That second double espresso can trigger this feeling. Neither dullness nor flightiness helps in the practice of Yoga. Progress comes when the mind is stable and focused.

Other conditions affect the functioning of your mind as well. Think about the last time you had a head cold or other illness; if you are like me, the thinking part of your brain just seemed to shut down. Even a low-grade fever can turn dreams into a cinematic scramble of epic nonsense. A psychotherapist once remarked that when you get into a stressful confrontation and the adrenaline starts pumping, your IQ drops by half! And think how excitement affects you. It's hard to imagine sustaining intense and stable awareness at the moment of a great victory or a crushing defeat. What about the impact of sexual arousal on our ability to think and reason? It is difficult to remain steady.

We have all experienced mild, temporary bouts of depression, perhaps brought on by stressful work or home conditions that suddenly seem just too much to bear. The emotional stress of feeling trapped robs the mind of creative thought, leaving us unable to figure our way out of the simplest of dilemmas.

A friend with a high-tech desk job once remarked that he envied the man doing physical labor, because he assumed the labor tired only the body, leaving the mind active and alert. Anyone who does hard physical work knows that this is not true: the mind has to drive the body, and when the body is exhausted, so is the mind.

So illness, stress, exhaustion, and even excitement, rooted in the body, have readily apparent and powerful effects on the mind, and deeply affect our ability to practice the concentration and meditation techniques of serious Yoga study. The ideal Yoga diet boosts the health and vitality of the body so that one has the energy to practice, the stability of mind to concentrate, and the clarity of inner vision to recognize and welcome the voice of the inner emotional-spiritual body.

*Yoga and Diet
in the Classical Texts*

For the most part classical Yoga texts emphasize the role of diet in advanced practices; for the beginner who just wants to do a few asans for limbering and relaxing, diet can be important but is not critical for success. However, if the student is motivated to attempt more advanced breathing, concentration, and meditation techniques, diet becomes more important. The classical texts all stress moderation of intake and the soothing, calming effects on the mind of a carefully designed diet.

The *Hatha Yoga Pradipika,* an ancient handbook of Yoga, says, "Moderate diet means pleasant, sweet food leaving free one-fourth of the stomach." The *Shiva Samhita,* a classic Sanskrit exposition of traditional Yoga practices, suggests avoiding acids, astringents, pungents, salt, mustard, bitter things, foods roasted in oil, and much eating (overindulgence, or the ancient sin of gluttony). Foods or categories recommended are clarified butter, milk, sweet foods, and betel nut without lime. This text also suggests that smaller, more frequent meals are beneficial.

The *Gheranda Samhita,* another classical Sanskrit text in the form of a dialogue between a legendary sage and an aspiring student, hints at a more practical approach. The sage says strong-tasting foods (which to us means highly palatable foods) are so attractive that they draw the mind to them. Food becomes a distraction. A blander diet retrains the mind, over time, to facilitate introspection. The following foods are recommended: rice, barley, wheat, and legumes (peas, beans, and lentils); and a wide variety of fruits and vegetables, particularly leafy vegetables. A general description of pure, sweet, and cooling food, filling only half the stomach, rounds out the recommendations. You can see the principle of moderation at work again. My teacher Rama explained that one-half of the stomach should be filled with food and one-fourth with water, leaving one-fourth for air.

Modern Yogis often follow these much older traditions. All three of my teachers, Sivananda, Rama, and Lakshmanjoo, were vegetarians who strictly followed the classical teachings just outlined. Rama and Lakshmanjoo, both of whom I knew well, were particularly insistent on freshness; no leftovers! All three adhered to the belief that turning away from meat, poultry, and fish was the best way to start serious Yoga practice.

THE YOGA VEGETARIAN DIET

As you can see, Yoga philosophers throughout the ages have recommended the lactovegetarian diet as most suitable for building health and creating a bright, stable frame of mind. In today's terms the Yoga diet is best described as a modified lactovegetarian diet, plant-based with the addition of dairy products and a few unfertilized eggs. My teacher Rama said that historically Yogis avoided eggs because they were available only from the wild and therefore were usually fertilized. He saw no reason to avoid eggs from modern supermarkets, which are all unfertilized and so acceptable. However, modern dietary guidelines urge restraint because of eggs' high cholesterol content; after all, one jumbo egg may contain more than an entire day's recommended maximum intake of 300 milligrams of cholesterol.

Moving Toward a Vegetarian Diet

Some experts claim that the easiest path to success is a total and abrupt change of diet, but we feel that for most people, a more gradual approach is needed. My students seem to experience less disruption to their lives by changing just a few habits at a time. If you are considering changing your diet, try these recommendations.

- *Cut back on junk food.* Please keep in mind that although a grilled American cheese sandwich on white bread with a side of French fries is technically vegetarian, that is not the sort of diet we are talking about here! Try replacing junk with nutritious substitutes: fruit juice for sodas, whole-grain cookies for those made with refined flour, roasted soybeans instead of peanuts, baked chips instead of fried, and so on.
- *Increase the number of servings of whole-grain cereals, breads, and starchy vegetables such as potatoes, corn, and winter squash.* These foods provide the feeling of "fullness" that signals us we have had enough. Their complex carbohydrates fuel our bodies and minds for many hours.
- *Add more fruits and vegetables.* Nine out of ten Americans do not eat the recommended number of servings of these vitamin-, mineral-, and fiber-rich foods. Focus on dark green leafy vegetables such as kale, mustard and turnip greens, and Chinese cabbage. The cruciferous vegetables—cabbage, cauliflower, broccoli, and Brussels sprouts—are cancer preventers. Go for darker fruits such as mangoes, melons, and apricots, as well as dried fruits, to maximize your nutritional intake.
- *Replace meat, poultry, and fish entrees with legumes (peas, beans, and lentils),* including soy products, such as tofu, fortified soy milk, and soy-based meat substitutes, such as bacon, burgers, hot dogs, sausages, and sandwich slices. All these are low- to no-fat alternatives to high-fat meat, fish, and poultry.
- Use fat-free or low-fat dairy products as often as you can. Milk, yogurt, ricotta, and cottage cheese are all available in low-fat or fat-free varieties. Try the new fat-free alternatives to sour cream, cream cheese, half-and-half, and even hard cheeses such as cheddar. I am still looking for a hard cheese substitute with full flavor, but the fat-free products now available are adequate for some cooking uses, such as cheese sauce or a grated topping for a baked dish.

THE AMERICAN YOGA ASSOCIATION FOOD PYRAMID

Nearly everyone is familiar with the U.S. Department of Agriculture (USDA) Food Guide Pyramid, which suggests how to build your daily diet in terms of servings of different food groups. First published in 1992, it has a visual format that effectively com-

PERCENTAGE OF TOTAL DAILY CALORIES

SOURCES AND PORTIONS

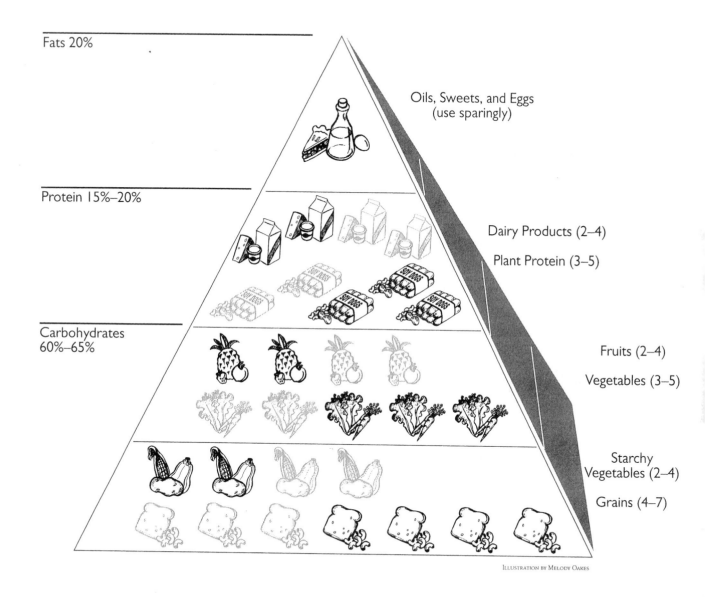

Fats 20%

Protein 15%–20%

Carbohydrates
60%–65%

Oils, Sweets, and Eggs
(use sparingly)

Dairy Products (2–4)

Plant Protein (3–5)

Fruits (2–4)

Vegetables (3–5)

Starchy
Vegetables (2–4)

Grains (4–7)

ILLUSTRATION BY MELODY OAKES

THE AMERICAN YOGA ASSOCIATION FOOD PYRAMID
A Guide for Healthy Vegetarian Nutrition

municates the idea that a healthy diet consists of an abundance of the foods grouped at the bottom, fewer of the foods at the next level, and so on.

We have modified the USDA pyramid to represent our guidelines. Ours is a whole-food vegetarian diet, with plenty of dairy food and an occasional egg. It is low-fat because the dairy products, particularly the milk, yogurt, and cottage cheese items, are all fat-free. Recommended fats are usually in the form of olive, canola, or peanut oil for cooking and salad dressings, and supplemental flaxseed oil for essential fatty acids.

Levels 1 and 2—Carbohydrates: 60 to 65 Percent of Total Calories

Starting from the two lowest, widest levels, our modified pyramid emphasizes whole grains, fruits, and vegetables. We recommend from 11 to 20 servings daily of these healthy, energy-producing foods. If this seems like a lot, consider the relatively small serving sizes noted for each category. There is naturally some overlap between levels. Starchy vegetables would usually include peas, beans, and lentils, but we have listed them in Level 3 as meat substitutes because of their protein content.

GRAINS (BREAD, CEREAL, RICE, AND PASTA): 4–7 SERVINGS

One serving is 1 slice of bread, 1 ounce of ready-to-eat cereal, or ½ cup of cooked cereal, rice, or pasta.

- Stick to whole grains whenever possible.
- White-flour baked goods, such as doughnuts, cakes, pies, cookies, croissants, and pastries, are too high in fats and sugars to be anything except a rare treat.

- There are many great whole-grain hot cereal varieties available, oatmeal being the most popular. Reach for them instead of the more common highly refined ones.

STARCHY VEGETABLES (POTATOES, CORN, AND WINTER SQUASH): 2–4 SERVINGS

One serving consists of ½ cup of cooked potato, corn, or squash. One medium potato, either white or sweet, is a serving. A large ear of corn on the cob is usually pretty close to a ½-cup portion.

- Potatoes and corn are traditionally loaded up with fats: butter, margarine, sour cream, cheese (or cheesy sauce), so learn to make some adjustments. I like lemon juice and salt on baked potatoes, and some of my friends enjoy plain yogurt in place of sour cream. Baked beans or vegetarian chili as a topping gives you an extra protein serving as well. French fries are too fatty to call good food; they're especially high in trans–fatty acids, which raise cholesterol.
- If corn is fresh, nothing needs to be added, unless you are used to a little salt. Winter squash is usually baked with a little sweetener, such as real maple syrup or liquid fructose, or it can be added to soup.

VEGETABLES (SALAD, DARK GREEN LEAFY, CRUCIFEROUS, AND SO ON): 3–5 SERVINGS

One serving consists of 1 cup of raw leafy vegetables, such as salad greens, or ½ cup of cooked or chopped raw vegetables. Some people enjoy vegetable juice, but it isn't actually a whole food. If you really like it, limit your intake to 6-ounce servings.

- If you like dressing on salad (often I prefer just a little vinegar or lemon juice and seasoning), there are many low-fat recipes available.
- Dark green leafy vegetables are especially rich sources of vitamins and minerals, so try to include them several times weekly.
- Always ask for "dressing on the side" when dining out so you can use less.

FRUITS (MELONS, CITRUS FRUITS, APPLES, PEARS, PEACHES, BANANAS, GRAPES, PLUMS, BERRIES, DRIED FRUITS, AND SO ON): 2-4 SERVINGS

One serving consists of a medium apple, banana, or orange, or ½ cup chopped, cooked, or canned fruit. Fruit juice, like vegetable juice, is not a whole food, has little fiber, and is high in rapidly absorbed sugars. If you can't get along without it, stick to 6-ounce servings and be sure what you buy is 100 percent juice, not merely a "juice drink" with lots of added sugar and water.

- Eat whole fruits whenever possible. Avoid processed fruit products, such as fruit canned in heavy syrup.
- Citrus, melon, and berries (especially blueberries) are highest in antioxidants.

Carbohydrates come in two forms: the first is digestible, consisting mainly of complex starches and simple sugars; the second is indigestible fiber. Many dietary guidelines recommend eating less sugar; one good reason is that for some people simple carbohydrates can make blood fats rise, perhaps even raising cholesterol levels. Some experts suggest that overconsumption of sugars also brings on diabetes.

Don't forget that alcohol of all kinds contains concentrated amounts of sugar.

Complex carbohydrates from whole foods are less efficiently converted to and stored as fat, are more filling, and are lower in calories per volume than comparable processed and refined foods. High-carbohydrate foods are also usually high in fiber. A high-fiber diet is associated with lower weight and also contributes to long-term cardiovascular health by lowering blood fats, cholesterol, and insulin levels. Fiber alters the mix of bacteria in the gut and provides needed bulk in the colon.

By eating a wide variety of the recommended servings of fruits, vegetables, whole grains, and legumes, you will automatically increase your fiber intake. Most foods contain a combination of soluble and insoluble fiber, and both are important to good health. Foods richest in soluble fiber, which is the type believed to help reduce serum cholesterol, include oat bran, oatmeal, and rice bran. Most other whole-grain foods are good sources of insoluble fiber. Always read labels to be sure you are getting a maximum amount of fiber in combination with low fat and cholesterol. Beans, peas, and lentils are also good sources of soluble fiber. To help eliminate some of the gas problems associated with eating these foods, discard the soaking water and rinse beans before cooking to eliminate the indigestible sugars they produce. Soak canned beans in water for 1 hour and discard the water. If you are unaccustomed to eating a substantial amount of high-fiber foods, increase your fiber intake gradually. And be sure to drink plenty of water (6 to 8 glasses per day) to avoid constipation. Citrus fruits, strawberries, and high-pectin fruits such as apples are also high in soluble fiber.

I would like to note that there is a common misconception among healthy-minded people that brown rice is vastly superior to white rice. Brown rice becomes white by a polishing action that removes a very thin layer of bran from each grain. When cooked, however, both forms contain essentially the same amount of protein. White rice is a little higher in calories, but the only significant difference seems to be magnesium content, which is lower for white rice. However, neither type of rice is a rich source of this mineral. White rice is usually the only type available at Indian, Chinese, or Mexican restaurants, and when you really need a break from the kitchen, I believe you can enjoy it guilt-free.

Level 3—Protein: 15 to 20 percent of Total Calories

The third level of the pyramid consists of protein and dairy foods. (Remember that the grains and other foods in Level 1 provide a bit of protein, too, especially when complemented by dairy or legume protein. See below for more on complementary proteins.)

DAIRY PROTEIN (MILK, BUTTERMILK, CHEESE, AND YOGURT): 2–4 SERVINGS

One serving consists of 1 cup of milk, buttermilk, or yogurt, and 1 ounce natural (2 ounces if processed) cheese. I always look for fortified fat-free milk, which is skim milk with extra nonfat milk solids added to improve taste and protein and calcium content (as much as 40 percent).

- I like to use hard cheeses for flavoring when I cook, but otherwise I stick to other dairy foods because the higher saturated fat and cholesterol content just aren't worth it.

- I often use fat-free versions of half-and-half, cream cheese, sour cream, and whipped topping, especially for festive occasions.
- Many people, as they age, have less of the digestive enzyme lactase, and so experience bloating, discomfort, and diarrhea after consuming too much lactose-rich dairy food. However, almost everyone can tolerate small amounts of lactose, for instance, the amount in an 8-ounce glass of milk. If lactose is a problem for you, try lactase enzyme supplements and lactose-reduced milk products.

PLANT PROTEIN (LEGUMES, TOFU, MEAT SUBSTITUTES, SOY MILK, NUTS, AND SEEDS): 3–5 SERVINGS

One serving consists of ½ cup cooked beans, peas, or lentils; 3 ounces tofu; 1 cup soy milk; 1 egg; 2 tablespoons peanut butter; 1 ounce nuts; 1 veggie burger or soy wiener.

- Most Americans eat about twice as much protein as they need, which increases calcium excretion and stresses the kidneys. Here is a simple way to determine how many servings of protein foods you need every day: multiply your weight in pounds by 0.4 if you are sedentary to moderately active, by 0.5 if you are very active, or by 0.75 if you need to build muscle. According to this formula, a 150-pound moderately active woman needs about 60 grams of protein daily. Each serving of dairy or plant protein listed earlier includes 6 to 14 grams of protein. The table on page 178 lists the protein content of some common foods; if you are interested in a more complete list, consult one of the reference books listed in the Resources.

- Soy products are now readily available in major supermarkets, and most people are familiar with soybean curd (tofu), a staple food of Asia; it is a bland, cakelike, high-protein food that can be barbecued, scrambled, sautéed with vegetables, boiled, or baked. When processed with calcium, as it usually is, tofu is a great source of this essential mineral as well as protein. Although nearly 50 percent of tofu's calories are from fat, the fat is predominantly unsaturated, and at least one major brand has introduced a reduced-fat version.

- Enriched soy milk is readily available at supermarkets as well as health food stores; it consists of soybeans, rice or cane syrup, and water to which calcium and vitamins have been added to mimic the consistency of milk. Try it on your favorite whole-grain cereal or blended with ice and fresh or frozen fruit for an excellent smoothie.

- I use many "fake meat" products, such as wieners, burgers, Canadian bacon, and deli slices. They are certainly healthier for you than the meats they mimic because they are usually fat-free. Even if you are not a vegetarian, you will benefit from adding some of these foods to your diet; a "veggie" hot dog or slice of "veggie" bacon as a snack will quell hunger pangs just like the real thing.

- Nuts and seeds are excellent sources of healthy oils and antioxidants as well as protein, but they should be eaten in moderation because of their high calorie content. Peanuts and cashews are the highest in protein. Try adding English walnut halves to tossed salads or cereal.

COMPLEMENTARY PROTEINS

It is now well accepted that plant foods can adequately meet the protein needs of both adults and children. All plant foods contain essential amino acids, though they are often in short supply. Some plant foods, soy in particular, are amino-acid rich. You are probably familiar with the idea of complementary proteins, which means that different plant foods, when combined, are equivalent to animal protein. This combining effect works even when the foods are consumed at different meals. For example, the bean tortilla you eat at lunch will complement the oatmeal you ate for breakfast. Here are a few other ways to combine protein groups:

- *Grains plus dairy protein:* breakfast cereal with milk; yogurt with a whole-grain, low-fat muffin; pasta with low-fat ricotta; a hard cheese sandwich made with whole-grain bread

- *Grains plus peas, beans, and lentils:* brown rice mixed with beans or tofu "crumbles" in a casserole or as a stuffing for peppers, tomatoes, or squash; whole-grain toast with pea or lentil soup; Mexican tortillas (wheat or corn) and rice with beans; whole-grain corn bread with bean chili; the classic Indian combination of rice with dal, a lentil; Chinese dishes that combine tofu, a soy legume, with rice

- *Peas, beans, and lentils plus seeds:* Middle Eastern hummus is chickpeas with sesame paste (tahini is ground sesame seeds). Make your own without oil for a really low-calorie dip or spread. Roasted soybeans may be combined with sunflower or pumpkin seeds for a great protein snack

PROTEIN CONTENT OF SOME COMMON FOODS

Food	Protein
1 cup fat-free yogurt	13.0
1 ounce Swiss cheese	7.0
1 cup nonfat milk	8.0
1 egg white	3.5
1 cup low-fat buttermilk	8.0
½ cup dried beans	7.0
1 fat-free soy "hot dog"	11.0
1 cup brown rice	5.0
1 tablespoon peanut butter	4.0
1 cup soy milk	8.0
½ cup roasted soy nuts	34.0
½ cup tofu	10.0

Level 4—Fats: 20 Percent of Total Calories

This category includes fats and oils, sweets, and eggs.

FATS AND OILS

Use fats and oils sparingly. Fats are vitally important elements of our diet that aid in the absorption of the fat-soluble vitamins (A, D, E, and K) and provide energy reserves, insulation, and protection for the body. You might be thinking, If fat is so important to health, why do nutritionists always talk about the danger of fat in the American diet?

The problem lies in the types and quantity of fat that most Americans consume. Many health problems, such as obesity, diabetes, some forms of cancer, and heart disease, are associated with excessive intake of fats, particularly the saturated fats found in meat and butterfat as well as in hard margarine, commercially fried food, and most processed foods. A few saturated fats come from plant sources, such as palm, palm kernel, and coconut oils, and cocoa butter. Some sources estimate that the average American consumes over 40 percent of his or her daily caloric intake in fat—that's 900 to 1,350 calories a day. Nutrition experts recommend limiting our total fat consumption to the more appropriate range of 10 to 30 percent (we recommend 20 percent) and reducing the amount of saturated fat to below 5 percent.

- The majority of fat calories should be from monounsaturated fats, as found in olive, canola, and peanut oils.
- Unless you are really rigid about fat-free dairy products, you will get a small amount of butterfat daily. Nuts and seeds can contribute appreciable amounts of polyunsaturated fats as well.
- It is important to improve the balance of EFAs (essential fatty acids) in your diet. Most people get too much of the omega-6 fatty acids—from common vegetable oils such as cottonseed, sunflower, and safflower—and too little of the omega-3 fatty acids, which are much rarer. Canola, soybean, and flaxseed oils are the only relatively rich sources of linolenic acid that can be metabolized into omega-3 fatty acids. For most people, 1 teaspoon daily of flaxseed oil is sufficient.

SWEETS

Use sweets sparingly. The USDA recommends limiting sweets to between 6 and 12 teaspoon equivalents of sugar daily, if for no other reason than simple calorie overload. Most cakes and pies include about 6 teaspoons per serving, and fruit and flavored yogurts also weigh in at 6 teaspoons, while chocolate shakes and soft drinks contain about 9 teaspoons. The food with the highest sugar content is fruit drink, with 12 teaspoons for a 12-ounce drink. For a more comprehensive list of added sugar in common foods, check out the USDA's Food and Nutrition Information Center web site (www.nal.usda.gov/fnic).

EGGS

Use eggs sparingly. Eggs are a great source of protein, but the yolks are very high in fat (about 6 grams) and cholesterol (about 250 milligrams). The American Heart Association recommends limiting cholesterol intake to 300 milligrams daily. Egg whites, however, are fat- and cholesterol-free and a great source of protein.

How Many Servings Are Right for You?

Here are some very general rules to follow. If you are older, small in stature, inactive (meaning sedentary), a chronic dieter, athletic (because of higher metabolic efficiency), female, or have a low metabolic rate, adjust your serving quantities down. If you have a hard time maintaining your ideal weight, lean toward the low end of the ranges of servings.

By contrast, bigger (by weight) and younger people, or those who are moderately to very active, can afford to eat more servings. Men tend to have higher metabolic rates and can tolerate more servings than women.

How to Prepare Foods for Maximum Nutrition

Fruits are best when fresh and raw, because antioxidants are lost during cooking. Vegetables should be eaten raw, steamed, or quickly sautéed to preserve nutrients; frying, boiling, and baking tend to reduce nutrient value. However, there are some exceptions: exceptionally woody vegetables such as carrots release more nutrients, especially minerals, when cooked. Try boiling or steaming them. Grains usually must be boiled or baked for digestibility. Generally speaking, the longer you cook fresh foods, the more vitamins and other phytochemicals they lose. That said, the loss is often balanced by greater availability of minerals, provided the cooking water is retained; add it to soups or sauces for its flavor as well as nutritional value.

Cooking over a hot open flame can produce some pretty harmful toxicants. Smoking, broiling, grilling, frying, and roasting, all methods of cooking with intense heat and limited oxygen, form potent mutagenic chemicals in the surface layers of foods. This is especially true of meat, poultry, and fish, but any fatty or protein food (cheese or tofu, for example) can be affected. If you indulge in these cooking methods, try using lower-than-recommended temperatures and avoid scorching.

See Resources for cookbooks and nutrition books to supplement this information.

SUPPLEMENTS

Vitamin and mineral supplements cannot replace whole foods, each of which is a vastly complicated storehouse of yet-to-be-discovered chemicals that may be important to health. Our whole-food vege-

BEST FOOD SOURCES OF VITAMINS AND MINERALS

*H*ere is a simple rule of thumb for getting the vitamins you need from your diet. Eat whole grains for **B complex,** fresh fruits and vegetables for **vitamins A** (as beta-carotene), **C, E, and K.** Apricots, mangoes, citrus fruits, bananas, melons, and dried fruits are all excellent sources. The vegetables with the highest vitamin content are always the most colorful ones: a few examples are dark green leafy vegetables, such as spinach, chard, collards, mustard, and kale; and carrots, tomatoes, and colorful peppers. All members of the cabbage family, such as broccoli, cauliflower, Brussels sprouts, and cabbage itself, along with winter squash, are also vitamin-rich.

All **B-complex vitamins** are included in whole-grain products except for **B$_{12}$,** which is found naturally only in milk, eggs, meat, fish, and poultry. Vegetarian or reduced-meat diets need a reliable source of B$_{12}$, such as multivitamin supplements, fortified breakfast cereals, and soy beverages. Eggs supply most of the other B-complex vitamins, as do many fruits and vegetables. **Vitamin D** is added to milk and is formed on the skin by sunlight.

Iron-rich foods include beef and pork; you'll find moderate concentrations of iron in prunes, apricots, spinach, beans, tofu, blackstrap molasses, nutritional yeast, and wheat germ. However, the iron content of fortified cereals dwarfs all other sources. For example, a serving of Total brand cereal contains 18 milligrams of iron, which is 100 percent of the recommended daily intake. Younger people, especially premenopausal women, need the full amount of iron, but older men and women should be okay with up to 10 milligrams daily. Vegetarians need to be sure to include these iron-rich foods and to use a multivitamin-mineral supplement with iron. But the message isn't simply the more, the better. Iron is a powerful oxidizer that can damage vitamin E and possibly even oxidize LDL cholesterol, which may damage arteries.

Zinc is needed for growth and development, but it is much more difficult to obtain, with only beef, pork, and shellfish being good sources. Wheat germ, garbanzo beans, and lentils are the best of the rest, but in order to get the recommended 15 milligrams, you would need to eat nearly 1½ cups of wheat germ! A mineral supplement that includes the recommended amount of zinc makes good sense, and most multivitamin-mineral supplements do.

Calcium is highest in dairy foods: milk, yogurt, and cheese. Include plenty of low-fat and fat-free varieties in your diet. Other good sources include tofu (if processed with calcium sulfate; read the label), fortified soy milk, and some dark green leafy vegetables (especially turnip and mustard greens, kale, and Chinese cabbage). Vegetarians absorb more calcium from foods, perhaps because of their lower fat levels or higher levels of vitamin C in the gut. Unless you commit to eating at least four servings per day of high-calcium nonfat dairy foods, take a calcium supplement in place of each high-calcium serving you miss.

Magnesium is an important part of calcium metabolism, affecting nerves and muscles in artery walls. It also reduces the risk of diabetes. Whole grains and beans are the best sources, especially if they were grown in magnesium-rich soils. I take a calcium supplement that includes magnesium (about 1:3 or 1:2 magnesium-to-calcium ratio) for convenience, because the amount of magnesium in most multivitamin-mineral supplements is inadequate and I have no way of knowing the magnesium content of the soil my food is grown in.

Trace minerals are difficult to track, but a diet that includes a wide variety of unrefined foods, such as whole grains and fresh fruits and vegetables, will provide your body with most of the trace minerals it needs. The single exception is **selenium.** Add 200 micrograms (*micrograms, not milligrams*) selenium to your supplement list for protection from prostate, lung, and colon cancers as well as antioxidant protection for your arteries. Most multivitamin-mineral supplements contain this amount.

tarian diet supplies a vast range of naturally occurring vitamins, minerals, and other compounds that science is just now learning about, such as carotenoids, flavonoids, and phytoestrogens, which you can't find in a supplement tablet. In fact, vitamin and mineral supplements contain only a handful of these essential nutrients, so it is best to eat a wide variety of foods prepared in ways that preserve the naturally occurring vitamins and minerals. That way you'll also avoid potential chemical excesses and imbalances. See the sidebar for the best food sources for vitamins and minerals.

It is a fact, however, that Americans are generally not eating enough of the right foods. Too many of us eat too much junk food and too many high-fat and high-sugar restaurant meals, and then try to repair the damage with sporadic efforts at highly restrictive dieting. Because of this, we do recommend a few safe and effective vitamin and mineral supplements as nutritional insurance.

Who Should Supplement?

- *Dieters:* Given that the majority of Americans are overweight, it may seem that everyone you meet is dieting. If you seriously restrict calories in order to lose weight, important vitamins and minerals may well be missing from your diet. Even a well-balanced diet can be lacking in adequate amounts because of restricted quantity and portion size.

- *Those at risk for heart disease:* Many experts believe that the body's ability to safely process cholesterol is overwhelmed by diets high in cholesterol and saturated fats. All aspects of diet affecting the body's ability to re-

pair damaged arteries, to lower circulating levels of cholesterol and triglycerides, and to protect healthy artery tissue are important, and safe and effective nutritional supplements ensure their optimal functioning.

- *Those at risk for gastric cancer:* Not surprisingly, the alimentary canal, which is in direct contact with food, is most affected by our dietary choices. Supplementing vitamins C, E, and beta-carotene, as well as calcium, may reduce the risk of oral, esophageal, stomach, and bladder cancer, and extra calcium reduces the risk of colon and rectal cancer. Isoflavones, found in soy products, stimulate natural killer cells throughout the body to resist cancer growth. In fact, vegetarians have reduced risk for developing cancer at all major sites.

- *Those at risk for arthritis:* The common antioxidant vitamins A, C, and E and selenium are low in the fluid of arthritic joints, possibly impairing the regeneration of healthy tissue. Some sufferers also benefit from the B vitamins, especially niacin, pantothenic acid, B_6, and folic acid. Glucosamine and chondroitin have been shown to relieve symptoms of arthritis.

- *Older people:* The older population most at risk for arthritis, cancer, coronary heart disease, hypertension, and diabetes is also most likely to be overweight. I say it's never too late to do something about that and urge those readers to restrict food intake to lose weight. Older people often have irregular eating habits and do not eat a well-balanced diet, whether they're dieting or not. Depression, loneliness, lack of appetite, loss of the senses of taste and smell, and denture problems can all contribute to a poor, inconsistent diet. Absorption of vitamins and minerals can also be impaired in older people. Older women often need extra vitamin D and calcium for protection from osteoporosis.

- *Women:* Women have special nutritional needs, starting with calcium and vitamin D to prevent osteoporosis. Lower levels of these nutrients increase the risk of developing arthritis, a condition that affects twice as many older women as men. Women of childbearing years usually do not get enough folic acid, which increases the risk of neurological birth defects and also increases levels of homocysteine, which is damaging to the arteries. Doctors customarily prescribe vitamin and mineral supplements for pregnant and lactating women, whose nutritional requirements are pronounced.
- *Strict vegetarians (vegans):* Those who eat absolutely no animal products (that means no dairy products or eggs) are unlikely to get adequate amounts of vitamins D, B_2, and B_{12}, calcium, iron, and zinc. They should at the very least consider supplementation.

Select a Well-Balanced Multivitamin-Mineral Supplement

A comprehensive multivitamin-mineral supplement is a simple and relatively inexpensive choice. You do not need to spend a lot of money on a supplement. The cheapest "store" brands are often as well balanced and effective as the premium brands. I usually go to large retailers, where the price is lowest. The basic multivitamin-mineral supplements can cost as little as ten cents per day or as much as fifty cents a day, though there is no discernible advantage to buying the high-priced options.

The vitamin and mineral compounds in all supplements are manufactured by a small group of multinational corporations, such as ADM. "Natural" vitamins are no better in quality than other choices you'll see alongside them. Many supplements include additives such as herbs and enzymes, but they contain these compounds in such tiny amounts that they can do you no real good. The only quality issues for supplements are (1) nutrient content (does the tablet contain the labeled amount?), (2) whether the tablet will dissolve properly, and (3) purity. Although there are no federal standards for vitamins, the letters "USP" on the bottle indicate voluntary compliance with the U.S. Pharmacopeia. Most major brands have this listing.

When I was eliminating artificial coloring from my diet to relieve symptoms of rheumatoid arthritis, I learned to buy uncolored brands or, if possible, I rinsed the superficial color coating off, leaving only the hard white shell on the tablets.

I usually take vitamin-mineral supplements after a meal for better absorption, and I take vitamin E and calcium at a different time of day than the basic multivitamin that includes iron. Calcium interferes with iron absorption, and iron may rapidly oxidize the vitamin E. Some experts suggest not taking vitamins and minerals at the same time as any prescription medications, so wait a few hours between to reduce the risk of interference.

The following name-brand recommendations for multivitamin and mineral supplements are adapted from the *Nutrition Action Health Letter* (see Resources), April 2000 issue.

FOR WOMEN

Centrum, Dr. Art Ulene's Nutrition Boost Formula for Men & Women, Kroger Complete Extra, One-Source, Rite Aid Whole Source, Safeway Select OmniSource, Spring Valley Advantage, Summit Complete, Twinlab Dualtabs, Walgreen's Ultra Choice, YourLife Super Multi-Vitamin.

FOR MEN

Dr. Art Ulene's Nutrition Boost Formula for Men & Women, Eckerd Daily Impact Senior, Rite Aid Whole Source Mature Adult, Safeway Select OmniSource Senior, Shaklee Vita-Lea without iron, Twinlab Dualtabs, YourLife Super Multi-Vitamin.

FOR OLDER MEN AND WOMEN (OVER FIFTY)

Dr. Art Ulene's Nutrition Boost Formula for Men & Women, Eckerd Daily Impact Senior, Rite Aid Whole Source Mature Adult, Safeway Select OmniSource Senior, Twinlab Dualtabs.

Supplemental Antioxidants and Minerals

The tablet size of the recommended multivitamin-mineral supplements is too small to include adequate amounts of several important nutrients, so please consider adding them separately. Extra amounts of vitamins E, C, and beta-carotene, along with calcium and magnesium, are useful to almost everyone, and countless studies have demonstrated their safety and effectiveness.

- For **vitamin A** it's best to depend on a diet rich in **beta-carotene**-containing fruits and vegetables, such as apricots, mangoes, cantaloupes, carrots, and sweet potatoes, and limit supplements to a *total* daily amount of 15,000 IU of vitamin A and beta-carotene combined. All good-quality multivitamin-mineral supplements contain 5,000 IU of vitamin A, so add 10,000 IU of beta-carotene daily to achieve the 15,000 suggested amount on days when you do not eat darkly colored fruits and vegetables.
- You need daily doses of 500 to 1,000 milligrams of **vitamin C** in order to saturate all the tissues. More than that is simply excreted. The best plan is to take 500 milligrams twice daily. Multivitamins usually contain only a small fraction of this amount.
- **Vitamin E** benefits seem to increase with daily amounts in capsule form up to 400 IU. Again, taking more does not increase the benefit. Multivitamins usually contain 30 to 60 IU.
- **Calcium, magnesium,** and **vitamin D** are all critical for bone health and often need to be supplemented. You need 1,000 to 1,200 milligrams calcium daily (in 300-milligram doses), and one-third to half that for magnesium. You may skip a dose for every meal that includes a serving of a high-calcium dairy product, tofu, or vegetable. Vitamin D is included in most multivitamins and added to many dairy products, so an additional supplement is not advisable.
- With these exceptions in mind, it is a good idea to limit your intake of vitamins and minerals to no more than 150 percent of the recommended daily allowance. Large amounts of some vitamins and minerals, particularly vitamins A and D, can be toxic.

Chapter 8

℘REGNANCY

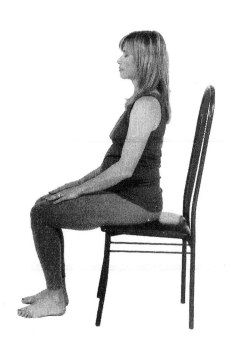

*D*uring pregnancy you and your body have a very special relationship. You are both working together for one purpose, which overrides all others: living healthily to produce a healthy baby. Instinctively your body knows what to do, and Yoga can help you support this special work.

A Yoga routine during the last six months of pregnancy is focused primarily on improving relaxation skills. This training will help relieve lower back pain and postural tension as your carriage changes with weight gain, and it will improve your ability to relax during labor and delivery. The simple routines also help strengthen your nervous system and increase joint limberness and strength. If you have begun a Yoga routine before your pregnancy, you will have an easier time maintaining it through your term, and the benefits will increase. Be sure, however, to shorten your routine as recommended in this chapter.

If you are planning to become pregnant, you can give yourself and your baby a head start by taking steps to improve your health right now. Try to improve your diet, get enough rest, learn techniques to help manage stress, and practice Yoga exercises to build a strong nervous system and lower back, improve circulation in your legs, and increase joint limberness. If you practice Yoga regularly, by the time you become pregnant, your routine will have become second nature, and it will be that much easier to continue. Practice meditation and breathing regularly. Imagine in detail what kind of baby you'd like to have. You and the prospective father can both do this exercise.

As soon as you suspect that you are pregnant, take a break and do not resume until the first trimester (three months) has passed. The reason for this precautionary measure is that in the first few months of pregnancy your body is working hard to establish a new hormonal balance. Yoga exercises, particularly those involving compression, have a powerful effect on the hormonal system that can obstruct or counteract the natural hormonal balance of pregnancy.

After the first three months you may resume a modified Yoga exercise routine as outlined in this chapter—assuming there have been no complications and your doctor approves. If your doctor suggests maintaining a secondary form of exercise during your pregnancy, discuss the possibilities with him or her; perhaps a mildly aerobic workout such as briskly paced walking or swimming to build overall fitness appeals to you. Most women are encouraged to keep up their regular levels of daily activity. However, keep in mind that starting a new exercise activity is not usually recommended in the middle of your pregnancy.

HELPFUL HINTS

As you practice your medically approved routine during the second and third trimesters, do only what is comfortable. You may find it increasingly difficult toward the end of your term to motivate yourself to exercise. Do not force it. Enjoy meditation and stillness.

Because of the increased levels of certain hormones during pregnancy, your joints will naturally become a bit loose. Be careful not to injure yourself: Pay attention to your kinesthetic sense (the awareness of where your body is in space) and move deliberately and slowly. If you normally run or participate in other vigorous exercise (and your doctor approves of your continuing), be especially careful; you don't want your good intention to stay

fit to end in a fall. Be aware that your center of gravity is changing also, which naturally affects your balance. Hold on to a sturdy chair or counter for extra support when doing standing exercises.

Breathing techniques can be done in any comfortable seated position. Use one or more pillows under your hips for extra height if you sit on the floor, in order to reduce strain on the lower back. You may also sit on the edge of a chair for breathing (see page 144 and all of Chapter 5 for more suggestions on proper posture and seat for breathing). Many women find that Yoga practice complements Lamaze training because of the emphasis on paced, focused breathing.

Some women report that meditation during pregnancy becomes more difficult as their mental and physical strength is depleted by the developing baby's needs. They describe the feeling as like a warm woolen cap fitted over their brain. It becomes much more difficult to achieve a quiet mind as the pregnancy develops. If this happens to you, shift your attention from achieving complete silence to the experience of complete physical and mental relaxation. Use the relaxation procedure as taught, but make it a process that you employ for the whole session. Concentrate on problem areas, such as the face, the stomach, and the shoulders, and focus on recognizing tension areas and relaxing the tension at will. This training can improve your concentration and ability to relax as you go into labor. A welcome plus is that your happy, calm, and relaxed attitude will produce a happy and relaxed baby.

Practice your relaxation/meditation lying down; sitting with your back against a straight chair or the wall; or seated with crossed legs. Experiment with one or more pillows under or between your knees, under your lower back, or under your head for additional comfort. You can lie on your side with a pillow under your head, one between your knees, and perhaps another under the side of your stomach. Any position that is comfortable for you is the position you should use.

YOGA ROUTINE DURING PREGNANCY

Many of the exercises that follow are illustrated elsewhere in this book. Never do inverted (upside-down) positions when you are pregnant because of the danger of air embolism. Compression poses are also not recommended, except the Baby Pose and the Diamond Pose. Exercises described previously are listed along with their page numbers; new exercises* (indicated with asterisks) are illustrated on the following pages.

Arm Rolls (p. 27)
Neck Stretch (p. 28)
Shoulder Rolls (p. 25)
Elbow Touch (p. 26)
Easy Bend (p. 31)
Full Bend (p. 32; Hold on to chair with one hand, letting the other arm relax. To guard against hyperextending the spine, do not stretch too far down in this exercise.)
*Supported Leg Lifts (p. 187)
*Baby Pose (p. 188)
Cat Breath (p. 87)
*Pelvic Rock (p. 188)
Foot Flaps (p. 99)
Diamond Pose (p. 109)
Easy Spine Twist (cross-legged; p. 105)
Easy Bridge (p. 119)
Alternate Toe Touch (p. 115 through the seventh month only)

Here is a six-week course that you can begin in the first week of your second trimester.

WEEK ONE

Complete Breath, standing (p. 150)
Arm Rolls
Neck Stretch
Easy Bend
Baby Pose
Relaxation and Meditation

WEEK TWO, ADD

Full Bend (if allowed)
Foot Flaps
Diamond Pose and Warm-up
Humming Breath (p. 152)

WEEK THREE, ADD

Standing Reach without arm stretch (hold on to chair with both hands instead)
Sit Between Feet (p. 189)
Pelvic Rock
Supported Leg Lifts

WEEK FOUR, ADD

Easy Spine Twist
Easy Bridge
Alternate Toe Touch

WEEKS FIVE AND SIX

Continue same routine

Supported Leg Lifts

Stand beside a chair, holding on to the back for support. Stare at one spot on the wall in front of you to help you balance. Keep breath relaxed. Lift one leg forward about three times (A), then to the side (B), then back (C). Keep foot flexed at all times to strengthen leg and increase circulation. Repeat on opposite side.

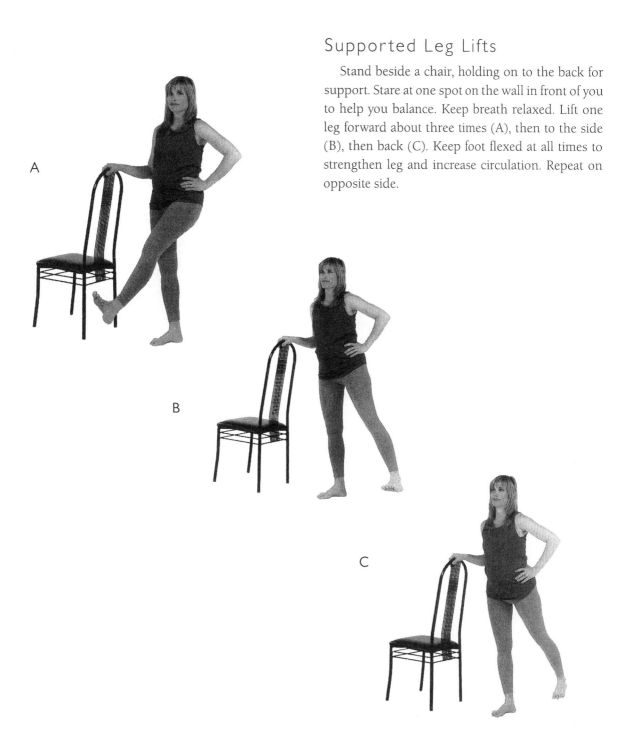

Baby Pose

Separate your knees a foot or more—as far as is necessary as your abdomen increases in size (A). If discomfort results from your head being below your heart, rest your head on your arms as shown here instead of resting your hands by your feet as shown in Chapter 4. If this pose becomes too uncomfortable (this is a normal occurrence), just relax for a few minutes in your favorite rest position.

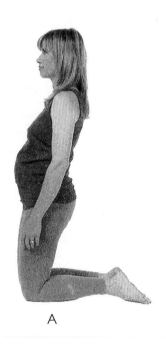

A

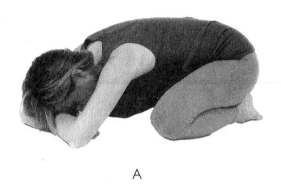

A

Pelvic Rock

This exercise, illustrated here as a kneeling pose (A), can also be done standing or seated on your feet. Its purpose is to strengthen and relieve tension in the lower back. Kneel with your back straight. Exhale, pulling your lower back and stomach in, making a straighter back without slouching. Then breathe in, letting your stomach relax, and arch the lower back forward (this movement is similar to the Cat Breath). Repetitions: 3.

Breathing

Your breathing routine will be enhanced by sitting between your feet, which will also help limber your hips and knees (A). Use one or more pillows under your hips for extra comfort. I recommend all seated floor poses for promoting flexibility and joint strength. Sit on the floor while watching television, reading, or playing with other children in the family.

The Complete Breath is your best technique for coping with stress at any time of day. It can be done standing, sitting, kneeling, or lying down. You can also practice the Complete Breath during many other daily activities, such as while waiting in the doctor's office. The Complete Breath can also be an effective sleep aid. The Humming Breath is a good focusing exercise to change your mood or relax when you're feeling jittery. Use the Laughasan (p. 153) to relax your facial muscles and change mood.

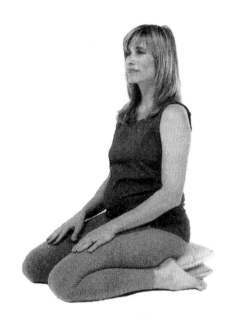

A

NUTRITION FOR PREGNANCY

Before you get pregnant, give your baby a healthy start by developing healthy eating habits for yourself. Make sure you are following a balanced and varied diet. Be particularly careful to reduce fats to recommended levels. Please see Chapter 7 for our nutrition suggestions for healthy adults. It is a great idea to meet with your physician and plan your pregnancy ahead of time. Healthy lifestyle changes can benefit your pregnancy plans too. If your vices include cigarettes, coffee, and cocktails, consider changing your habits now. Don't wait until you're pregnant.

If you are already pregnant, scrupulously follow the advised schedule for checkups with your physician. Your nutritional requirements are higher during this time, and also while lactating. Your physician will usually prescribe vitamin and mineral supplements. Carefully follow the instructions and dosage plans. It is particularly important to provide the growing baby inside you with enough B vitamins, especially folic acid and B_{12}. You'll need additional iron, calcium, and zinc as well. Some women find that adding a balanced B vitamin supplement helps to reduce the incidence of morning sickness.

As your baby grows, many of your organs, including your stomach, are subjected to extra pressure. If it is uncomfortable for you to eat normal-size meals, start eating several smaller meals a day instead. This will help by frequently replenishing your body with the nutrients that are important in coping with stress. Be very careful to plan your meals so that you do not eat junk food snacks that add empty sugar and fat calories. I recommend six small, balanced, and varied meals.

If you decide to nurse, we again recommend that you reduce the amount of Yoga exercise you do. Because of the strong hormonal changes brought about by Yoga asans, which may affect the composition of your milk, we suggest practicing only the following Yoga techniques while nursing:

Arm Rolls
Neck Stretch
Tree Pose (p. 74)
Sit Between Feet
Complete Breath
Relaxation and Meditation

Chapter 9

YOGA AND SPORTS

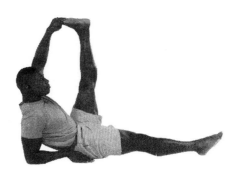

HOW YOGA HELPS IMPROVE SPORTS PERFORMANCE

The slow, controlled, and relaxed movements of Yoga asans can be complementary to active sports and will help improve your performance.

How Asans Help

Practicing a Yoga asan routine every day will build a reserve of flexibility and strength that will keep you in shape, encouraging you to exercise more often, stay fresher, and recover faster. Yoga can also help by balancing the muscle groups that are underused in your favorite sport. Strength-flexibility imbalances are the greatest causes of injury. Runners, for example, strengthen the muscles in the backs of their legs, but without stretching exercises, those muscles will tighten more and more. This chapter will give you a general routine to keep you in the best condition, and it includes suggestions for stretches that work best for different sports.

How Breathing Helps

Use Yoga breathing exercises to enhance your sports performance by increasing your stamina. The Belly Breath is especially helpful because it teaches you to keep your stomach muscles relaxed while you are exercising, which helps to prevent side stitch. Using the Complete Breath before competition will focus your mind and increase your concentration.

*How Relaxation
and Meditation Help*

A daily practice of Yoga relaxation and meditation can train you to become more aware of your body. If you are competitive, relaxation training can help you cope with precompetition anxiety so that your performance is not hampered.

YOGA TECHNIQUES FOR WARMING UP AND COOLING DOWN

Whether you are a competitive athlete or work out periodically to condition your heart and lungs, you can benefit from using Yoga asans to help you warm up and cool down.

Warming up is important: it's a way of telling your body that you are about to demand more work from it. If you and your body work as a team rather than at odds, you will both enjoy your activities a lot more. Learn your body's weak points, its likes and dislikes, its fears and comfort levels, and then gently coax it toward your athletic goals. Take the time to understand and encourage your body rather than forcing it or "whipping it into shape."

Many experts agree that the *static* or relaxed holding stretches of Yoga are ideal for warming up before and cooling down after a strenuous workout and actually work better than the bouncy, *ballistic* stretches that many inexperienced athletes use. Muscles automatically contract when they are stretched near their limit. It's an involuntary reaction, something our bodies do to avoid muscle tears. A static stretch allows the muscle to relax gradually and then stretch even further without injury. However, if the muscle is pushed to its limit with quick bounces, it retains the contraction and is much more vulnerable to tearing, both as you're stretching and later, as you work out.

Cooling down after your workout is just as important as warming up beforehand. Many people who allocate adequate warm-up time tend to leave out or skimp on cooling-down time. While it is true that your body will eventually recover by itself, it will take longer unless you spend a few minutes helping the process along. Be sure to take adequate time to cool down.

During a workout your muscles contract and your blood pressure naturally rises as your heart pumps faster to supply muscle cells and tissues with needed oxygen. If you end your workout abruptly, your blood pressure falls rapidly, slowing the flow of much-needed oxygen to fatigued muscles. In addition, you may experience dizziness, nausea, or light-headedness. To avoid these symptoms, keep moving for a few minutes after a workout—walk around awhile, then start some stretches to keep oxygen flowing, flush out metabolic wastes, and start any cell repair work. First stretch the muscles that were used the hardest during your workout, then end with general stretches.

Following are a few suggestions for using the exercises described earlier in this book—along with some new ones—to help you get the most from your sports activities. If you like, add one of the specialized routines to your general daily sports routine.

DAILY YOGA ROUTINE FOR IMPROVED SPORTS PERFORMANCE

Shoulder Rolls (p. 25)
Elbow Touch (p. 26)

V-Raise with Bent Leg

In the V-Raise position, with your head tucked under and legs straight, bend one leg as you shift your weight to the straight leg, pressing that heel toward the floor to stretch the back of the leg (A). Hold for a few seconds, breathing gently, then repeat on the opposite side.

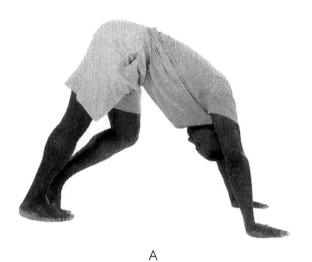

A

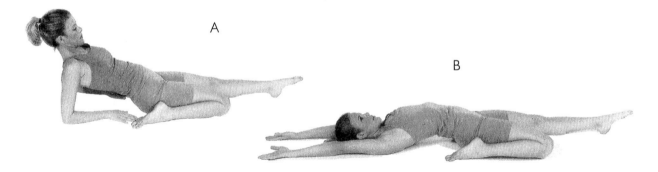

A

B

90-Degree Stretch

Begin in a seated position with your legs out-stretched. Bend your right leg at the knee so your foot and toes rest near your right hip. Stretch your legs apart as far as possible—eventually you want your right thigh to be perpendicular to your outstretched left leg. Now lean back on your elbows (A), or as far as possible, and hold, breathing gently, for several seconds. If you are very limber, you may be able to lie completely back (B). Repeat on the opposite side.

Lunge

Assume a modified lunge position: left foot forward, right leg back, and right knee resting on the floor. Place your fists on either side of your left foot; your left fist will actually be in back of the left foot, with your elbow tucked under your bent knee (A). Hold the position for a few seconds, breathing gently. Repeat on the right side. When you can do this without strain, try lifting your back knee off the floor (B). To intensify the stretch and extend it to the groin muscles, bend farther toward the floor so that you are resting on your elbows instead of your fists (C).

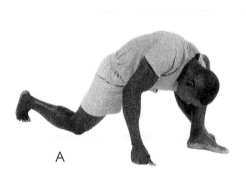

A

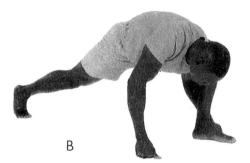

B

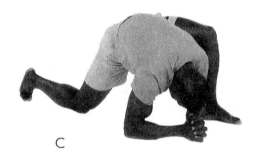

C

Thigh Stretch II

In this variation, start in Thigh Stretch position (p. 96) but tuck the toes of the back leg under. Breathe in to a count of three as you look up and stretch forward, lifting the back knee off the floor (A); then breathe out to a count of three as you straighten both legs, tucking your head toward your front leg as far as possible and pushing the heel of your back leg down toward the floor (B). Repeat on the opposite side. Repetitions: 3 on each side.

Hamstring Stretch on Back

Begin seated with your legs extended in front of you. Lean back on your right elbow, bend your left leg, and grasp your toes with your left hand. Slowly straighten your left leg as far as possible without strain and hold for several seconds, breathing normally (C). Repeat on the right side.

A

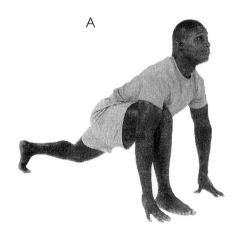

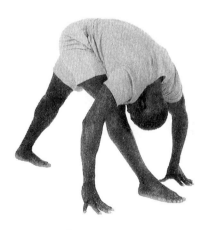

B

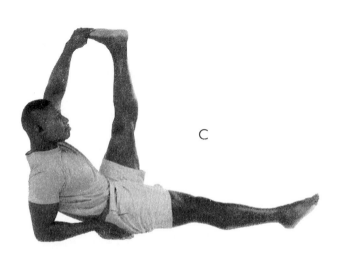

C

Suggestions for Your Favorite Sport

FOR BICYCLING

To stretch chest and stomach, and to strengthen lower back, add

Side Triangle (p. 70)
T Pose Knee Bends (p. 81)
Camel Pose (p. 95)
Cobra Pose (p. 137)
Arm and Leg Balance (p. 86)
Pigeon Pose (p. 97)

FOR RACQUETBALL, TENNIS, AND SIMILAR SPORTS

To strengthen knees and lower back, stretch inner thighs, improve respiration, and extend range of motion in shoulders, add

T Pose Knee Bends (p. 81)
Side Triangle (p. 70)
Twisting Triangle (p. 71)
Full Triangle (p. 68)
Hero Pose Variation (p. 92)
Sun Pose Variation (p. 85)
Easy Balance Twist (p. 65)
Bow Variation (p. 89)
Airplane Series (p. 133)

FOR WEIGHT LIFTING

To stretch all muscle groups, especially backs of legs, chest and stomach, and upper and lower back, add

Full Triangle (p. 68)
Side Triangle (p. 70)

Twisting Triangle (p. 71)
Lunge (p. 194)
Pigeon Pose (p. 97)
Seated Sun Pose (p. 100)
Alternate Seated Sun Pose (p. 103)
Cobra Pose (p. 137)
Spine Twist (p. 106)
Pelvic Twist (p. 118)
Bow Pose (p. 138)
Plow Pose variations (p. 127)
Hamstring Stretch on Back (p. 195)

FOR SWIMMING

To improve range of motion of shoulder joints, strengthen lower back, stretch upper back and ribs, and improve respiration, add

Dancer Pose (p. 76)
Alternate Triangle (p. 69)
Easy Balance Twist (p. 65)
Sun Pose Variation (p. 85)
Side Triangle (p. 70)
Bow Variation (p. 89)
Pigeon Pose (p. 97)
Cobra Pose (p. 137)

FOR GOLF

To strengthen lower back and improve flexibility of spine, especially laterally, add

Spine Twist (p. 106)
Alternate Triangle (p. 69)
Twisting Triangle (p. 71)
Dancer Pose (p. 76)
Knee Squeeze (p. 113)
Cobra Pose (p. 137)

FOR SKIING

To strengthen knee joints and lower back, and to stretch ankles, thighs, and backs of calves, add

Side Triangle (p. 70)
Cobra V-Raise (p. 90)
Seated Sun Pose (p. 100)
T Pose Knee Bends (p. 81)
Ankle Stretch (p. 94)
Thigh Stretch II (p. 195)
Pigeon Pose (p. 97)

FOR WALKING AND RUNNING

To stretch backs of thighs and calves, tops of ankles, and fronts of thighs, add

Dancer Pose (p. 76)
Lunge (p. 194)
Thigh Stretch II (p. 195)
Ankle Stretch (p. 94)
Camel Pose (p. 95)
Seated Sun Pose (p. 100)
Alternate Seated Sun Pose (p. 103)
Hamstring Stretch on Back (p. 195)

Chapter 10

STRESS MANAGEMENT

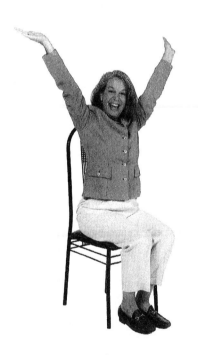

Life is never entirely free from stress, but often it seems that everyone else has less of it than we do. Some people are less affected by stress because of their outlook on life: they have learned that by maintaining their health and strength and adjusting their point of view, they can perceive the stresses of life as challenges and opportunities rather than hindrances. Such people do not automatically meet new or unexpected events with despair, anger, or dread. Because of their balanced outlook, they effectively reduce the time and effort it takes to recover from a stress reaction.

If you do not recognize yourself in this description, perhaps this chapter can help you change the way you react to the stress in your life. Each person's life has its particular tensions. Some are manageable; some are not. You cannot eliminate the experiences that cause you stress, but you can change your reaction to it. For example, if you habitually respond to traffic delays with anger and frustration, we can show you how to substitute a more appropriate and productive response. Simple Yoga techniques practiced during the course of a day can help with physical and emotional stress responses such as anxiety, depression, muscle tension, insomnia, and irritability.

When someone mentions stress, what is the first thing that comes to your mind? If you are like most people, it is probably something unpleasant. We have learned to associate stress with the worst of everything—pressure at work, difficult relationships at home, short tempers, furrowed brows, antacids, illness, and so on. What most people overlook is the fact that some stressful events can signal positive change. Indeed, a life without any stress would be very dull. A promotion, a wedding, a move into a new home—these are usually happy events that also involve some stress.

Yoga's view is that the body reacts the same way to "good" stress and "bad" stress. It views all stressors as demands—usually only temporary but sometimes extended—for more work and energy output. Recalling a past stress can also create a demand, because the mind reactivates the initial physical reaction—feelings of fear, excitement, anger, pain, anxiety, and anticipation. We carry a library of painful events in our memories to dip into at will. Even an imagined or anticipated stressor can trigger a physical reaction. In fact, emotional stressors can be more debilitating than physical ones, because we are socially conditioned not to act on them.

For example, if you walk into the street and see a truck approaching at high speed, your body immediately and automatically responds by triggering your muscles to get you quickly out of the way. Once you are safe, your body's systems start to return to normal. But difficult personal or professional relationships may prompt intense emotional reactions that you are unable to resolve right away. You may not have the opportunity to express your feelings or to work out the tension physically until much later (if at all), leaving the negative stress reactions to accumulate in your body and mind. Muscular tension, obsessive mental replaying of a stressful confrontation, and strong emotional reactions are common signs of internalized stress reactions.

Communication with your physical and emotional-spiritual bodies becomes especially important when you are trying to become more stress resistant. In this chapter we will show you how to recognize your body's reactions to stress and offer techniques for eliminating this debilitating and exhausting physical syndrome. Yoga can help you recover from the demands of life stresses faster and at the same time give you the training for healthy responses.

Schedule some of the following stress-reduction techniques into your daily work routine. Mark them on your appointment calendar or post a small reminder above your work station or at home on the bathroom mirror or refrigerator. Remember that the effects of Yoga practice are cumulative, so the more you practice the techniques, the more effective they will be.

THREE STEPS TO GREATER STRESS RESISTANCE

1. Learn to Recognize Your Body's Signals

Here are some examples of signals your body may send you when it is under stress:

- *Physical:* Frequent headaches, migraine headaches, numbness in extremities, unusual amount of blinking or yawning, rapid heartbeat, rapid breathing, nervous tics, teeth clenching, nausea, insomnia, sighing
- *Perceptual-cognitive:* Loss of perspective (making a mountain out of a molehill), forgetfulness, misperceptions (failing to hear or see accurately), inattentiveness or distractibility (daydreaming, poor concentration), replay of stressful events
- *Emotional:* Blowing up/loss of temper, high or low irritability (either everything or nothing bothers you), unexplained or prolonged depression, crying for unknown reasons

● *Behavioral:* Nervous habits (foot tapping, pen clicking, and so on); sudden changes in diet; clumsiness; increased use of substances such as alcohol, caffeine, tobacco, and sugar

States of mind are often mirrored in the body. Expressions such as "Grin and bear it," "Keep a stiff upper lip," and "the strong, silent type" describe a common stress response: tightening facial muscles, especially along the jaw. Although these expressions describe reactions to stress and pain, most cultures ironically hold these responses as models of self-control and strength.

Can you think of other expressions that illustrate the way we respond to stress?

He's a pain in the neck. Translation: I tighten my neck and throat muscles to avoid saying how I really feel about him.

I am petrified she's going to get angry with me. Translation: I am so afraid of her response that my brain can't send the right signals to my muscles for me to move naturally; I feel stiff.

He makes my blood boil. Translation: Since I don't dare tell him what I think of his actions, my emotional reaction produces a visceral one: my blood pressure and pulse rate go up.

You make me sick! Translation: Interactions with you trigger such anxiety that my stomach tenses.

I'm all keyed up about tomorrow's meeting. Translation: I am so frightened of the meeting that my muscles are tight and tense as if I were bracing myself for a physical attack.

Which parts of your body react most quickly to stress? Take a few minutes right now to write down how your body reacts to stress.

2. Learn Which Techniques Are Most Effective in Modifying Your Stress Reactions

All day long your body stores muscle tension. Perhaps you sat or stood in one position for too long; you couldn't express your feelings; you sat slumped at your desk; or you felt anxious. We're not meant to be as inactive as most of us are. Inactivity coupled with stored muscle tension compounds fatigue. In some ways the efficiency of modern office design exacerbates muscle tension. If you have only to swivel your chair to get from file cabinet to keyboard to telephone to copier to supply shelf to coffee machine, you'll miss out on opportunities to walk around, change your breathing, or stretch. Combine that sedentary condition with poor air circulation, uncomfortable chairs, and caffeine and junk food, and it's no wonder you are tired at the end of the day.

Did you know that you can use water to change the way you feel? Before you eat, wash your hands and sprinkle some water on your face, symbolically washing away any anxious feelings. After work (or at least sometime before bedtime) take a warm shower or bath. The heat will help relax your muscles. Imagine the water rinsing away the troubles and tensions that cling to you each day.

In mythology, water is often used to symbolize a change in consciousness. Water can be a daily reminder to broaden our outlook so that we don't waste energy on minor, unnecessarily stressful details that don't really matter in the long run.

Yoga exercises release stored muscle tension by gently pushing, stretching, and compressing muscle tissue, nerves, blood vessels, and the major organs. By performing a balanced series of movements regularly, you can reduce the amount of tension you take home at the end of the day. Plus, the extra circulation gets more oxygen and health-building nutrients to your brain, where they will help keep you alert. If you often feel sleepy and lethargic in the late afternoon, it may be the result of stiffened neck muscles that reduce blood circulation to your head.

Your Body's Target Zones

Here is a list of the major trouble spots for stored tension and the Yoga techniques that can best help. (See p. 204 for an all-around routine that combines a little of each of these four sets of techniques.)

1. NECK/UPPER BACK
   Shoulder Rolls (p. 25)
   Elbow Touch (p. 26)
   Neck Stretch (p. 28)
   Arm Rolls (p. 27)
   Standing Reach (p. 30)
   Easy Bend (p. 31)

Poor posture, repetitive keyboard work, hunching forward to see a computer monitor better, sitting in one position too long—all these fatigue the muscles in the upper back and neck, which react by tensing. Often this tightness reduces circulation to the head, which can result in tension headaches.

2. LOWER BACK
   Back Arch (p. 146)
   Folded Pose (p. 203)
   Knee Squeeze (pp. 38, 113, or 202)

Full Bend (p. 32)
Cat Breath (p. 87)

Work that requires a lot of standing or bending, poorly fitted furniture that does not support the lower back, as well as pathological problems—slipped, swollen, herniated, or degenerating disks—can cause aches and pains in the lower back. Lower back and hip inactivity can also contribute to impaired circulation and stiffness in the legs.

3. FACE/JAW/TEMPLE
   Lion (p. 153)
   Meditation (pp. 160, 206)
   Neck Stretch (p. 28)
   Folded Pose (p. 203)

There are dozens of tiny muscles in our faces, which we use to express all sorts of emotions; yet these muscles also tighten up easily, especially if we clench our teeth. Sometimes headaches result from this tension, which constricts the blood vessels in the head. These vessels respond by dilating, which is the real cause of the pain.

Note: If you often get pain in your temples, cheekbones, and bridge of your nose, you may have a chronic sinus condition.

4. ABDOMEN/CHEST
   Belly Breath (p. 149)
   Back Arch (p. 146)
   Seated Spine Twist (p. 202)
   Cat Breath (p. 87)
   Folded Pose (p. 203)

The abdominal area is probably the most important of all. Tensing the muscles of your stomach, abdomen, and rib cage prevents you from breathing deeply and completely. As you have probably read already in Chapter 5, there is a direct connection between the relaxation of your breath and the state of your emotions.

Note: If you experience frequent, severe, or chronic pain in your abdomen or chest, your stress reaction may be masking an underlying treatable condition. Consult a physician before attempting any of these exercises.

Following are a few exercises that can be done in a chair, in street clothes. You learned standing or floor versions of these exercises earlier in this book. These instructions indicate that you should begin in standing or kneeling positions, but most can be done just as easily seated in a chair. Here are a few extra exercises.

Seated Spine Twist

Sit forward on the chair with your feet flat on the floor. Place your left hand on your right knee. With your right arm, hold on to the back, side, or seat of the chair, whatever is most comfortable. Look forward and breathe in to a count of three, then slowly breathe out to a count of three as you turn toward your right, pulling with both hands to twist your spine as far as possible without strain (A). Hold your breath out for a count of three, then breathe in and relax as you return to the front. Switch sides. Repetitions: 1 to 3 each side.

Seated Knee Squeeze

Sit forward on the chair with your feet flat on the floor and arms hanging at your sides. Breathe in as you lift your left knee up toward your face. Grasp the knee with both hands and hold your breath in while squeezing the knee toward your chest as far as you can (B). Hold your breath in for a count of three. Now release and breathe out to a count of three as you return the leg to the floor. Repeat with the right knee. If you have injured or arthritic knees,

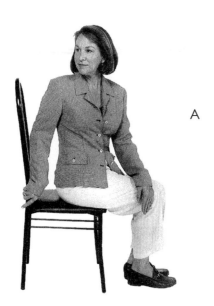

A

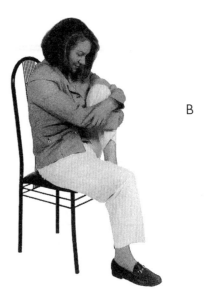

B

grasp your thigh just behind the knee instead. Repetitions: 3 on each side.

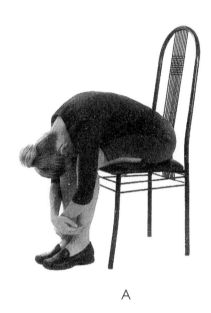

A

Folded Pose

Sit with your hips touching the back of the chair, feet flat on the floor. If your feet do not reach the floor, put a book under them. Separate your knees slightly. Lean forward, using your hands on your knees as a support. If you are comfortable, rest your chest on your knees, letting your head hang between your knees and your arms hang down at your sides. Alternatively, rest your hands on your lower legs or feet (A). If this position is not comfortable, cross your arms on your knees and rest your head on your arms. Let your breath relax.

3. Make Time Every Day to Put the Techniques into Practice

ANYTIME ROUTINES
Practicing Yoga techniques at any time of day will help reduce the effects of accumulated muscle tension before they turn into headaches or stomachaches. No one has to know that you're doing these exercises! Think creatively about times and places in which you can squeeze in a few exercises to keep your body feeling relaxed and strong. Turn these mini-practice sessions into a habit—just like eating regular meals. Managing stress is important for your total well-being. Here are a few examples of exercises you've learned earlier in this book and how they can be adapted for everyday use.

At your desk
    Seated Spine Twist (p. 202)
    Shoulder Rolls (p. 25)
    Elbow Touch (p. 26)
    Folded Pose (this page)
    Seated Knee Squeeze (p. 202)
    Belly Breath (p. 149)
    Complete Breath (p. 150)
    Standing Reach (p. 30)
    Back Arch (p. 146)
    Arm Rolls (p. 27)

In the kitchen
    Leg Lifts (p. 36)
    Arm Rolls (p. 27)
    Easy Bend (p. 31)
    Alternate Triangle (p. 69)
    Standing Reach (p. 30)
    Neck Stretch (p. 28)
    Lazy Stretch (p. 32)
    Easy Balance Twist (p. 65)

Watching television
  Seated Spine Twist (p. 202)
  Seated Knee Squeeze (p. 202)
  Folded Pose (p. 203)
  Lion (p. 153)
  Elbow Touch (p. 26)
  Back Arch (p. 146)

In the bathroom
  Standing Knee Squeeze (p. 38)
  Easy Bend (p. 31)
  Cat Breath (p. 87)
  Tree Pose (p. 74)
  Lazy Stretch (p. 32)
  Back Arch (p. 146)

On business trips or vacation
  Easy Spine Twist (p. 105)
  Easy Bridge (p. 119)
  Full Bend (p. 32)
  Easy Cobra (p. 136)
  Baby Pose (p. 84)
  Cat Breath (p. 87)
  Standing Sun Pose (p. 82)
  Half Shoulder Stand (p. 124)

"KEEP MOVING" ROUTINE FOR ANY TIME OF DAY

This routine features exercises you can do at your desk. Photocopy this page and post it in a prominent place in your office or home.

Here are a few other ways to keep moving: Walk quickly up and down stairs or around the block; take a brisk walk to the supply room or to lunch; park at the far end of the parking lot and walk to your building entrance.

  Neck Stretch
  Shoulder Roll

  Elbow Touch
  Seated Spine Twist
  Back Arch
  Seated Knee Squeeze
  Standing Reach
  Lazy Stretch
  Folded Pose
  Foot Flaps
  Standing Knee Squeeze

STRESS AND DIET

No discussion of stress would be complete without talking about nutrition, because an adequate diet is essential to repairing the destructive effects of stress. Extreme stress depletes the body's reserves of nutrients. If these are not replenished regularly by a varied and balanced diet, the drain can, over time, result in stress-related illnesses such as high blood pressure, chronic infections, and inflammation.

In some ways our bodies haven't changed much over the many thousands of years we've been on this earth. When we face a threat—either real or imaginary—our bodies react instantaneously, readying us for combat (fight) or escape (flight). It all starts when the brain, through its sensory apparatus, receives and interprets environmental signals to mean that we're in danger. Messenger hormones carry this "red alert" signal throughout the body, triggering several reactions at once:

1. Blood pressure rises and pulse rate increases, in order to speed the messengers and nutrients along their way.
2. Blood sugar increases (drawn first from available proteins, then from carbohydrate stores) to provide instant energy if it is required.

3. As stress increases, your requirements for protein, B-complex vitamins, vitamin C, and calcium rise.
4. Bodily functions that are not absolutely necessary to meet this crisis (such as digestion) slow down.
5. Sodium and water are retained to prevent dehydration, and too much potassium may be excreted in the urine.

All this happens very quickly. The body is now ready to face the threat (even if the threat is only imaginary or emotionally triggered). It seems silly that all this happens when someone directs a sharp word at you. Nevertheless, the body does not distinguish among physical, emotional, and psychological threats; it reacts exactly the same way to all three.

When the threat is removed, the body goes into the second stage—resistance—in which it repairs damage and resumes normal functions. The nutrients that are used up during stress must be replenished. Protein, once it has been broken down to form sugar for energy, remains in your system as sugar; vitamin C, the B-complex vitamins, and minerals are excreted.

It is easy to see the importance of a healthy diet in meeting the constant demands of stress. Essential nutrients must be ingested in sufficient amounts to ensure adequate supplies—not only to respond to stress but also to support normal functions during our almost continuous resistance stage: repair, rebuilding, and growth.

The best way to protect yourself against depletion of these necessary nutrients is to eat more frequent, nutrient-dense meals without increasing overall calories. Five or six small meals are better than the three or four many of us eat: minimal breakfast, coffee and sweet mid-morning, fast-food lunch, large dinner. If six small meals are not feasible for you, or if you are unable to limit the amount of calories you take in at each meal, the next best thing is to have a good breakfast and lunch, a light dinner, and high-protein, low-calorie snacks between meals. Eat dinner early in the evening and avoid snacking later, so you'll be hungry for breakfast. Eating more of your caloric total earlier in the day helps your body to burn off some of the calories instead of storing them as fat. Do you eat more junk foods when you are very stressed? If so, you may be compounding your stress reactions with poor eating habits.

Enemies of a stress-resistant diet are caffeine, alcohol, excessive sugar, and processed and refined foods. Caffeine actually mimics some of the features of the stress reaction. Alcohol and sweets add empty calories that displace nutrient-rich foods. Processed and refined foods are stripped of the vitamin and mineral content you need to replenish reserves depleted by stress reactions. Substitute healthy snacks for caffeine and sugar so that your body can achieve and sustain a healthy blood sugar level. After work try practicing Yoga instead of using alcohol to restore emotional and physical balance. Besides its obvious physical dangers, alcohol dulls your sensitivity to what is happening in your body and mind—exactly the opposite effect from what is desired in Yoga: sensitivity, creativity, and courage.

BREATH: YOUR MOST PORTABLE STRESS MANAGEMENT TOOL

People often offer this piece of advice in stressful situations: "Sit down and take a few deep breaths and you'll feel better." It usually works, doesn't it? Do you know why?

You may have noticed how your breath changes when you get excited, tense, angry, or upset. You can also achieve a change in your mental state by consciously changing your breath. An anxious or disturbed mind (one ready for fight or flight) creates a vicious cycle of tight breath patterns and frantic thoughts. Knowing how to use Yoga breathing exercises can be your best—and most readily available—stress management tool. Breathing exercises can help you quickly recover from a stress event by helping you quiet anxious thoughts.

The Belly Breath (see p. 149) is the best way to change a stressed state of mind instantly. Sit or stand up straight. Consciously relax and push out your stomach as you breathe in; squeeze it in as you breathe out. Concentrate on the sound of the breath in the back of your throat. This simple technique can help you break the vicious cycle of stressed mind–stressed breath. You will probably notice a difference within a few minutes.

Many people who often have trouble sleeping at night find that practicing breathing exercises in bed helps them relax, stop thinking about the day's events, and get to sleep. Practice the Belly Breath, as slowly as possible without straining, and concentrate on the sound of your breath alone. Eating the right food can also help. Having a high-carbohydrate dinner and bedtime snack makes your body feel more relaxed and drowsy. Use the complete relaxation procedure (see Chapter 6) to help you go to sleep.

RELAXATION AND MEDITATION

Have you ever felt confused, frustrated, or angry after a stressful incident and later, when you were more relaxed and clearheaded, wondered why you had such a strong reaction to something so trivial? Your thinking patterns change when you are under stress. It's almost as if your mind reverts to a more primitive, reactive state and judges only in terms of survival. When you're stressed, it's hard to concentrate, you have less patience for interruptions, and you may find it difficult to be creative.

Sometimes there are simply so many things crowding into your mind that thoughts are jumbled and anxious. At these times, try drawing back from everything for a minute or two. Giving your conscious, physical mind a rest often allows your inner emotional-spiritual body to sort things out and let the important things come forward into consciousness.

Practicing daily relaxation and meditation as part of your Yoga routine can help by giving you a foundation for achieving a more stable outlook. Try to remember how you feel during meditation, when you are completely still and relaxed. You can reproduce this feeling any time during the day. You can also benefit from doing a shorter version of the meditation technique.

If you can find a quiet spot where you won't be interrupted—your office, a conference room, or even the bathroom—try a short meditation to welcome the support of your inner emotional-spiritual body. You will find yourself refreshed, calm, and ready to tackle the rest of the day with new energy and in-sight.

If you can, first wash your hands and sprinkle water on your face as you think of the water cleansing and removing stressful thoughts. Sit comfortably with your back straight, hands in your lap, and eyes closed (A). Take a few deep, full breaths, concentrating on the sound as you breathe in and out smoothly and evenly. Then let your breath relax into its normal pattern. Consciously relax your face, paying special attention to the tiny muscles around your eyes and the muscles of your jaws. Relax your shoulders, arms and hands, and stomach. Relax your legs and feet, the back of your neck, and your head. Feel your whole body go limp, but do not slouch: Keep your back straight.

For the next few minutes, try to be silent in your mind. Stop talking to yourself. You will notice emotions and problems trying to crowd into your awareness; concentrate on returning to a feeling of stillness. Melt into the silence; let it surround you and fill you up. Rest in it. After a few minutes, start breathing deeply. Stretch your arms and legs, and feel yourself filled with renewed energy and strength. Then you can go back to your work with full power.

Stress can work to your advantage. With an open mind and knowledge of appropriate Yogic techniques, you can view anything that life puts in front of you as a challenge instead of an obstacle.

A

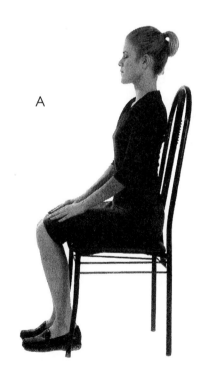

Chapter 11

YOGA PHILOSOPHY

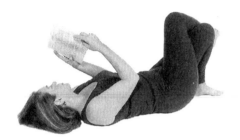

Yoga philosophy is best expressed by living example, not by talking about it. Anyone who writes on the subject of philosophy has a difficult task. It takes years for an individual to try to articulate the personal and historical philosophy of his or her life, and even then philosophy resists being put into words.

I certainly had no choice in my life. When a brilliant vision of light appeared in my bedroom, I had no idea what Yoga or the great philosophic background that it represented was. I only knew that after that time the thought of Yoga was always with me, and it continues to be to this day.

RAMA

I have referred to that brilliant vision of light in other books and writings, and introduced the great teachers who lighted my path. Sivananda was the first, although I saw him only in vision and knew him only through letters that followed. A few years after Sivananda died, my teacher Rama came to the United States. As he stepped down from the plane, he walked directly over to me and said, "Alice, I have come to get you." I had never seen him before, and, as a midwestern mother with two sons, I certainly was not looking forward to that kind of statement. I was filled with fright.

My book *The Light of Yoga* describes what happened to me after that: the long trip to India with Rama, living in the jungle, intense training and periods of silence, and the trek with him across India as he lectured and taught. However, I have never written about what happened after Rama's death in Cleveland, Ohio, in

1972. In the years before he died, Rama told me that his death would come very quickly and that afterward I was to go to Kashmir to search out his boyhood friend, the great scholar and teacher Lakshmanjoo. Rama told me, "He will take you through. Tell him I sent you."

I didn't want to talk about it. The thought of Rama gone from this life was too painful for me. However, I listened and remembered, and when Rama died I decided to try to find the great representative of the Shaivite philosophy, Lakshmanjoo, in Srinagar.

When my students in Cleveland realized I was going to keep my word, some of them wanted to come along. We had heard stories about the massive cave at Amarnath, high in the Himalayas. It is one of the great shrines of India. Many people feel that a visit to that place is the pinnacle of their lives, and all their families' lives, too. We decided to make the trek part of our trip.

A shepherd boy discovered the cave of Amarnath long ago. When he saw the huge opening, he walked inside to see an enormous lingam (phallus-shaped stone) made of ice formed by water dripping from the roof of the cave. He told his story of finding the "Abode of Shiva" to others, and over the centuries the pilgrimage to Amarnath became an annual event.

The lingam, a large ice pillar, waxes and wanes with the moon. It reaches its greatest height during the full moons of July and August. Thousands of people brave the terrifyingly difficult trip to the cave in order to receive the unseen mystical gift of spiritual philosophy. For most people the great beauty and strength of this philosophy begin when they salute the lingam in Amarnath. It is considered a life-changing experience: the culmination of the search for meaning in life. Thousands have died in the attempt. The high passes, some over 16,000 feet, and the unpredictable weather make for extremely dangerous travel.

This kind of pilgrimage demands people who are searching for something so important to their lives that they are willing to die in the attempt to know it. This describes my relationship with Yoga. This is philosophy as I see it: a driving freight train of thought that underlies everything you do. It never leaves. You can't get rid of it. It directs the whole epic of your life.

YOUR TWO BODIES

Yoga means "union." The word itself, as I stated earlier, comes from the Sanskrit *yug,* meaning "to join, to yoke together." Yoga philosophy states that individuals suffer from the pain of separateness, and that this pain drives them to seek relief. That relief is found in joining the two parts of oneself in a solid, impenetrable bond. These two bodies, which are discussed at great length in Yoga philosophy, are the outer, physical, "seen" body and the inner, emotional-spiritual, "unseen" body.

Yoga philosophy states that although the outer physical body is born and dies, the inner emotional-spiritual body does not die with it but continues on, through the death of the physical, taking another physical body again and again until the union is formed.

Once the union is complete, the result is called *realization.* In other words, realization means knowing who and what you really are. A more scholarly definition might be "the condition of being in full force." Lakshmanjoo talked about two states of existence: Being and Becoming, or subject and object.

The state of Being, or subject, corresponds to the inner, unseen, totally aware Self. The state of Becoming, or object, corresponds to physical experience, which relies on the senses and seems to be governed by space and time. *Object* also refers to mind, intellect, and ego. When the state of Becoming is ended and the state of Being is in full force, you rest in the inner body without separateness. You become complete, totally powerful, and unlimited. Lakshmanjoo emphasized that, through Yoga, object merges into subject. The inner being, the subject, expands to be all-inclusive, totally assimilating the outer physical existence.

All Yogic literature remarks on the fact that the physical body cannot be totally powerful without bonding with the inner emotional-spiritual body. Every text I have ever read, or have been fortunate enough to discuss with the great teachers in my life, states this fact clearly. The classical literature of Yogic philosophy describes many schools of Yoga, but joining the two bodies is always the ultimate goal.

The philosophy of Yoga cannot be learned intellectually; it can be learned only by emotional-spiritual experience. The personal experience of enlightenment and change comes from within as the steady practice continues. After Rama's death I continued with my study, hoping for that experience of realization. It is easy to write the word *realization,* but what does it mean? Yoga teaches not by words but by experience. I wanted that experience, and to strive for it I needed a teacher. I made plans to go to Kashmir as Rama had instructed me.

LAKSHMANJOO

You might laugh when I tell you that the first step I took was to sit down and write to one of Rama's devotees at an old address I had found in Rama's papers. I used to write many letters for Rama to devotees in Kashmir and India. In the letter I simply introduced myself and asked for guidance. I wrote, "I was Rama's student. He advised me to go to Kashmir to continue my practice. Having seen pictures of houseboats in Kashmir, I would like to rent one for the summer, possibly join the pilgrimage to Amarnath that summer, and then return home." I enclosed a check for three hundred dollars for a deposit to hold a suitable boat for our lodging and mailed it off to Krishan-Lal Kaul, Allied Motors, Srinagar, Kashmir, India. I didn't mention my search for Lakshmanjoo, because I felt that would begin when we got to Srinagar.

I received a quick response: "Yes, please do come. Your money is safe with me. Don't worry, just come. —Krishan-Lal." I had never met the man, yet he answered my letter warmly and encouraged me to go ahead with the trip. I was surprised and pleased and started to make plans. I fully believed I could live anywhere in the world. I had no idea what life was like in Kashmir but thought it couldn't be too much different than anywhere else. The food would be unfamiliar to us, and we'd have to be careful about the water we drank, but we could handle that. After all, I had lived and traveled with Rama across India for months on end. I was so naïve then.

We gathered our belongings, still planning eventually to reach Amarnath, and boarded a plane for Kashmir. Someday I will write a whole book about what happened, but for now just try to picture our little group landing in Kashmir. The flight was the only one scheduled for that week. The airport had one small runway and not much else. Still, lost in my American confidence, I headed for the exit. As I climbed down the staircase, a man came up to me with a picture in his hand. He said, "Excuse me, madam. Is this you? Are you Alice?" Indeed he had a picture of me in his hand—a very old and wrinkled picture, but it was me all the same.

I looked at him with astonishment and said, "Yes, that's me all right." He bowed and took my hand and said, "I have taken care of everything. Please come to my car." Well, what was I to do? I went. We drove to the city of Srinagar, which was a short distance from the airport. There was no conversation in the car. We watched and waited for information, but none was forthcoming until we drove through the gates of a beautiful house. We were ushered into a large room, where cushions were put down for us and tea was served. We were silent and grateful and waiting curiously to learn the reason for this surprising hospitality.

Krishan-Lal introduced his wife and family and then, leaning forward on his cushion, said, "Mother, we have been waiting for you all these years. Rama told us that you would come. He instructed us to build a house for you and to plant lots of apple trees in the yard because Americans like apples. He sent us this picture from America long ago and said we would be able to recognize you when you decided to come. We are overjoyed to see you here. We have put a bathroom next to your bedroom because Rama said that Americans like bathrooms next to their bedrooms. We are at your disposal. Now, if you would just tell us what you would like for supper, we will prepare it for you."

The whole scene was so unbelievable that I had trouble absorbing what was happening. I told him that we had looked forward to living on houseboats and would prefer that rather than putting him to the trouble of having houseguests. He was appalled, saying, "Mother, those houseboats are very dangerous for you. You would be safer here."

The whole afternoon and evening were overwhelming. I couldn't believe this was happening and, much to Krishan-Lal's dismay, eventually I insisted on heading for the accommodations I'd reserved. Krishan-Lal drove us to Dal Lake and installed us in houseboats and, after much consideration, left with the promise to have a man watch us all night. He would return in the morning. Eventually we did move into the house that had been prepared for us and lived there happily in the summer for many years.

That was my entry into Kashmir, and for the next twenty years we spent our summers studying in that place. We found the great Lakshmanjoo, and he accepted me as a student. So many memories are with me now as I write this from a quiet place in the woods of Florida. It was another world. Life in Kashmir was so different from life in the jungle with Rama. Nothing had prepared me for what was ahead. Every day was a new experience.

Lakshmanjoo was translating the massive works of Abhinavagupta, the legendary genius of the tenth century. The whole school of Shaivite philosophy (or the philosophy of Shiva) is still in existence thanks to Abhinavagupta's efforts. When Lakshmanjoo took me and Stephen Grant, one of the students who accompanied me, with him to the old library that overlooks Dal Lake, he pointed out a long list of names written on the wall. The list had a thick black line at the top, and above the line was Lakshmanjoo's name, all alone. He looked at us and said, "My name is above the line because all these philosophers are now dead and I am still alive. I am the last in the line." I have a picture of that chart here on my desk as I write these pages to all of you who have taken up this book to begin the long path that is Yoga.

In the summer of 1988 I arrived in Kashmir to find Lakshmanjoo in deep despair. The political troubles in the region at that time had resulted in two of his American students being deported on trumped-up charges. The loss of these precious relationships and the warlike atmosphere in his homeland were so troubling that he had lost interest in living. He had shaved his head (the traditional sign of impending departure from this world), had stopped eating, and was not speaking.

I refused to believe that this great teacher's work in the world was over, and I tried to think of a way to capture his interest. The best enticement, I knew, would be conversation about spiritual matters. Over the years he had told me many times how much he enjoyed talking to me about the inner aspects of Yoga. The year before I arrived in Kashmir, I had begun a lecture series on the ethical guidelines of Yoga, the yamas and niyamas. I begged Lakshmanjoo to tell me more about how these principles were described in the Shaivite philosophy.

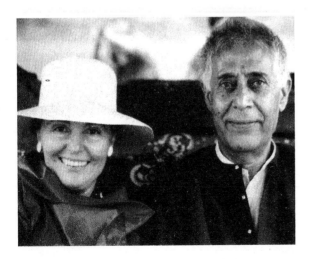

Little by little the subject drew him in, and he began to speak. His voice was weak and hoarse from lack of use, but day by day he grew stronger. We had brought a video camera with us, and he gave us permission to videotape many of our sessions. The transcripts of these and other conversations with Lakshmanjoo can be found in our books *Aspects of Kashmir Shaivism* and *Ethics of Yoga,* and in a three-volume videotape series (see Resources).

Lakshmanjoo died in New Delhi in September 1991—nineteen years to the day after the death of my Guru, Rama of Haridwar and Kashmir. I miss him terribly. I believe that his enlightenment will have a lasting effect on the world.

ETHICS IN YOGA

The first step to Yogic practice is the observance of personal ethics. I believe that my emphasis on the practice of ethics differentiates the American Yoga Association from most Yoga schools in the United States today. Ethical training must go hand in hand with all other Yogic procedures or the final product cannot be complete. Contrary to the way most Yoga classes are offered, we believe that ethical practice is the first consideration of the aspiring student, because it protects and guides the student in all life decisions. Practice of ethics produces a state of mind that is uncluttered by fear. Fear arises in the absence of ethical values and destroys meditative practice. A clear, ethical approach provides the greatest protection from fear.

Historically, students work to achieve mastery of these ethical guidelines before placing themselves in front of a teacher. Stories of the great *siddhas*—a name for those who achieve power—all tell of students spending long periods in self-examination, purifying the personality in order to face the Guru, the teacher they have chosen to take them through the difficult search for the Self. Yoga schools in the United States and some other countries usually do not speak of this essential preliminary work. Students simply decide that they want a class in Yoga and, without any preparatory training, start doing the asans and breathing and approach meditation with an attitude of entitlement: "I want the experience, I paid for it, now give it to me."

Ethics are the first two stages, or limbs, in the eight-stage classical Yoga system described in the book *Yoga Sutras*, which was written by the scholar Patanjali. There is some difference of opinion about the exact dates of his birth and death—estimates vary from 300 B.C.E. to A.D. 300. However, there is no doubt of his written contribution, which describes all the various schools of Yoga being practiced in India during his lifetime.

The eight limbs of classical Yoga are (1) *Yamas* (restraints), (2) *Niyamas* (observances), (3) *Asana* (exercises), (4) *Pranayama* (breathing techniques), (5) *Pratyahara* (withdrawal of the mind from the senses), (6) *Dharana* (concentration), (7) *Dhyana* (meditation), and (8) *Samadhi* (absorption). These are also described as the "eight stages of consciousness."

The first two stages, yama and niyama, are the ethical guidelines of Yoga. *Yama* means "restraint," and *niyama* means "nonrestraint" or "observance," and there are five yamas and five niyamas. What follows is a very brief description of each of these ten guidelines. If you are interested in learning more about the ethics of Yoga, they are fully discussed in my book *Yoga of the Heart* (see Resources). I would highly advise you to read that book if you are serious about Yoga study.

Nonviolence (Ahimsa) means not harming yourself, others, or the world around you. Many students overlook the fact that self-destructive behaviors such as overindulgence in alcohol or caffeine, drug abuse, and ignoring signs of fatigue are manifestations of self-violence. Nonviolence is first on the list because the other nine ethics depend upon it. For instance, lying to yourself or others (see Truthfulness) is also a form of violence.

Truthfulness (Satya) includes keeping your word to yourself and others and learning what is true about yourself. Lakshmanjoo told me that Truth can always be recognized because it is sweet.

Nonstealing (Asteya) applies not only to the obvious material things but also to more subtle things, such as stealing of time, attention, power, and confidence. An unsteady mind steals your ability to concentrate; fractured thought keeps you from reaching your goals.

Celibacy (Brahmacharya) has to do with observation of sexual preoccupation. Casual sex is a detriment. Love and sex have great meaning in Yogic practice; shallow relationships bleed your strength and fracture your life. Use Celibacy to appreciate what you want in relationships. Here is an easy way to practice Celibacy: for 5 minutes, preferably at the same time each day, try to clear your mind of sexual thought. Even practicing 5 minutes a day will change your life.

Nonhoarding (Aparigraha) means learning to simplify your life. Do not clutter your life with things to take care of that you do not want or need.

Purity (Shauch) is essentially about being 100 percent yourself: unfragmented, strong, and confident. Purity teaches you to reduce the quality of separateness in your life so that you can devote your full attention to what you want to achieve. Cleanse the mind and body with affection. Picture a new self, shining and clear, ready to approach the future bravely.

Contentment (Santosh) in Yoga means the ability to remain happily in the present moment. It brings an appreciation of happiness: a state of consciousness that is referred to as "wonder, delight, and astonishment."

Tolerance (Tapas) is usually incorrectly interpreted as harsh discipline or punishment of the body and mind. Tolerance is strength without violence in daily relationships. If you would like to practice Tolerance, choose something each day that you do not want to do and then do it happily, without injury to yourself or others.

Study (Svadyaya) is an important source of nourishment for your emotional-spiritual body. Spend some time each day reading inspiring writing that interests you and will help deepen your knowledge and experience.

Remembrance (Ishwara Pranidhana) is the constant recognition of the support that you receive from your emotional-spiritual body.

I've said it before, but it bears repeating: Yoga is not a religion. It has no creed. The student's personal Yoga practice is completely supported by personal ethics, which guide all behavior. Success in Yoga practice produces an extremely powerful ethical individual, one who is not dependent on society but in fact one on whom society depends.

Ethics allow a student to safely approach the inner emotional-spiritual body without harm, while protecting the outer physical body from self-destructive practice. The *Bhagavad Gita,* the great handbook of heroes, states, "Yoga is skill in action." The dedicated student soon finds balance and fulfillment in correct practice, learning to use the tools of ethics in every life situation.

Start practicing ethics by observing how much they are already a part of your daily life. Post the list of ethics where you will see it every day—on your refrigerator or bedroom mirror. Choose one ethic from the list and concentrate on it for a period of time: perhaps a week, a month, or even a day. Try to keep track of all the little ways that ethic asserts itself in your everyday affairs. You will be surprised at how often the issue you've chosen comes up in daily life. Make a conscious effort to change your actions and reactions to reflect the principle you are trying to put into practice. Doing this will also help to expand concentration in your daily life. Keep a journal or list of daily successes and failures, and watch your confidence grow as you practice.

Patanjali recommends the implantation of the opposite thought; for example, when a violent thought comes up, it can be replaced by a loving thought. This practice improves the power of mental focus. There is an old Buddhist saying: "As a man thinks, so he becomes." The more you think about and envision yourself becoming what you want to be, the more likely you are to reach that goal. The practice of ethical behavior will open new channels in your thought and create conscious behavior patterns to replace old, destructive habits.

I would say the most important quality that blooms with the practice of ethical standards is the ability to change. Change, usually so difficult as one gets older, becomes easy and delightful. Each day's decisions result from a simple formula: "If it fits my ethics, it's okay with me. If not, I'm out of here!" When you practice ethics this way, a clear path of behavior easily emerges. You feel strong, powerful, and happy with yourself.

Ethical practice will help you to take responsibility for your life picture. Strength and happiness can be within your grasp. Enjoy your voyage of self-discovery and learn how to delve deeply into your innermost self. Yoga will expose you to your many inner levels. First, with the gradual quieting of the mind in meditation, you can learn to bypass surface emotional turbulence and observe what lies beneath. As your concentration and observation skills improve, you begin to notice the patterns of your mind and the composition of your personality. You can start to experience the myriad possibilities that lie within your grasp.

If we could put the philosophy of Yoga into one word, that word would be *transformation*. Yoga enables you to transform yourself into what you want to be. Think of it as self-realization on the installment plan. You will begin to enjoy the experience of the present moment in everyday life. Yoga changes your life so that you are never bored. You can gain the happiness of knowing that you are on your way to achieving the goals you have set for yourself, whatever they may be. The treasures that wait for you along the way are the richness of experience, the warmth of friendship and love, the excitement of challenge, and the wonder of discovery.

Glossary

Agni Kriya—An advanced breathing exercise, introduced in Course 3, involving manipulation of the diaphragm while the breath is held out.

Ahimsa—Nonviolence, one of the five yamas, or restraints, which are the first of the eight stages of classical Yoga.

Ajna Chakra—A state of consciousness in which intuitive wisdom resides; represented in the body by the spot between the eyebrows.

Aparigraha—Nonhoarding, one of the five yamas.

Asan, or Asana—A position, posture, or movement in Yoga exercise.

Asan Point—In practicing asans, the point at which, after the body is correctly positioned and the breath held momentarily, the mind goes into silence.

Asteya—Nonstealing, one of the five yamas.

Bandha—A lock, or tightening, of particular muscle groups.

Bee Breath (Bramari Breath)—A breathing technique introduced in Course 2 in which fingers close off the sensory organs and the breath is exhaled as long as possible with a *zzz* sound.

Belly Breath—The introductory breath exercise, which teaches use of the diaphragm through emphasizing movement of the lower abdomen.

Brahmacharya—Celibacy, one of the five yamas.

Bramari Breath—See Bee Breath.

Complete Breath—A breath exercise of even inhalation and exhalation that involves all respiratory muscles.

Dharana—Concentration, the sixth of the eight stages of classical Yoga.

Dhyana—Meditation, the seventh of the eight stages of classical Yoga.

Easy Breath—A breath pattern that is relaxed and nonmanipulated.

Ekagrata—The ability to focus the mind voluntarily on an object without interruption for extended periods of time.

Hinduism—The major religion of India.

Humming Breath—A breath exercise that involves a short inhalation and long exhalation while making a humming sound.

Ishwara Pranidhana—Remembrance, one of the five niyamas, or observances.

Kapalabhati—An advanced breathing exercise introduced in Course 2 involving a period of short bellows breaths followed by a deep exhalation, inhalation, and an extended, silent exhalation.

Kashmir Shaivism—A school of Yoga philosophy that recognizes the essential unity of everything in the universe.

Kinesthetic sense—The awareness of where your body is in space.

Lingam—A phalluslike symbol of the creative force of the universe; called Shiva in Yoga philosophy.

Mantram—A sound that is repeated by Yogis to produce a change in consciousness.

Meditation—A state of complete silence and inner awareness.

Metabolism—The systems of the body involved in the production and utilization of energy.

Mulabhanda—A lock, or tightening, of the rectal muscles.

Neti—A nasal cleansing technique using warm salt water.

Niyamas—Five observances (Purity, Contentment, Tolerance, Study, and Remembrance), which together are the second of the eight stages of classical Yoga.

Om—A mantram used before meditation to help the practitioner experience silence.

Patanjali—A scholar who lived sometime between 300 B.C.E. and A.D. 300 who wrote down all the systems of Yoga in India in his time in a treatise called the *Yoga Sutras*.

Pranayama—The breathing techniques of Yoga.

Pratyahara—The withdrawal of the mind from the senses, an essential first step in meditation; the fifth of the eight stages of classical Yoga.

Samadhi—Absorption, the eighth of the eight stages of classical Yoga.

Santosh—Contentment, one of the five niyamas.

Satya—Truthfulness, one of the five yamas.

Shauch—Purity, one of the five niyamas.

Svadyaya—Study, one of the five niyamas.

Tapas—Tolerance, one of the five niyamas.

Tidal volume—The amount of air that is moved into and out of the lungs when in a resting state.

Vital capacity—The total amount of air that can be forcibly exhaled.

Yamas—The five restraints (Nonviolence, Truthfulness, Nonstealing, Celibacy, and Nonhoarding), which together are the first of the eight stages of classical Yoga.

Yoga—From the Sanskrit *yug,* meaning "to join together" or "to yoke." A system of techniques to enable the joining of the physical and emotional-spiritual bodies.

Yogi—Strictly speaking, one who has attained Yoga, or union of the two bodies, but used commonly to refer to anyone who practices Yoga techniques on a committed basis.

Resources

The following is a list of recommended reading on Yoga practice and philosophy, plus books and helpful web sites on diet and nutrition, focusing on healthy vegetarian nutrition. Books and tapes produced by the American Yoga Association are described on pages 221–224.

YOGA PRACTICE AND PHILOSOPHY

Shri Aurobindo. *Letters on Yoga.* 3 vols. Pondicherry, India: Shri Aurobindo Ashram, 1971.

The Bhagavad Gita. Many translations available. Choose one that is complete.

Campbell, Joseph. *The Hero with a Thousand Faces.* Princeton, N.J.: Princeton University Press, 1949.

Campbell, Joseph. *The Masks of God.* New York: Viking Press, 1962.

Campbell, Joseph. *The Mythic Image.* Princeton, N.J.: Princeton University Press, 1974.

Daniélou, Alain. *Yoga, the Method of Reintegration.* New York: University Books, 1955.

Eliade, Mircea. *Patanjali and Yoga.* New York: Schocken Books, 1975.

Eliade, Mircea. *Yoga: Immortality and Freedom.* Princeton, N.J.: Princeton University Press, 1958.

Iyengar, B. K. S. *Light on Pranayama.* New York: Crossroad, 1981.

Iyengar, B. K. S. *Light on Yoga,* New York: Schocken Books, 1965.

Swami Sivananda. *The Science of Pranayama.* Divine Life Society, 1978.

Swami Swatmarama. *The Yoga of Light: Hatha Yoga Pradipika.* Commentary by Hans-Ulrich Rieker. New York: Herder and Herder, 1971.

Taimni, I. K. *The Science of Yoga.* Wheaton, Ill.: Theosophical Publishing House, 1961.

Yogananda, Paramhansa. *Autobiography of a Yogi.* Los Angeles: Self-Realization Fellowship, 1977.

Zimmer, Heinrich. *The King and the Corpse: Tales of the Soul's Conquest of Evil.* Princeton, N.J.: Princeton University Press, 1957.

Zimmer, Heinrich. *Myths and Symbols in Indian Art and Civilization.* Princeton, N.J.: Princeton University Press, 1946.

DIET AND NUTRITION

Blonz, Ed. *The Nutrition Doctor's A-to-Z Food Counter.* New York: Penguin Books, 1999.

Bricklin, Mark. *Prevention Magazine's Nutrition Advisor.* Emmaus, Pa.: Rodale Press, 1993.

Chelf, Vicki Rae. *Cooking with the Right Side of the Brain.* Garden City Park, N.J.: Avery, 1991.

Clark, Nancy. *Nancy Clark's Sports Nutrition Guidebook,* 2nd ed. Champaign, Ill.: Human Kinetics, 1996.

Davis, Adelle. *Let's Get Well.* New York: Harcourt, Brace & World, 1965.

Davis, Adelle. *Let's Have Healthy Children.* New York: Harcourt Brace Jovanovich, 1972.

Davis, Adelle. *Let's Stay Healthy: A Guide to Lifelong Nutrition.* New York: New American Library, 1983.

Loma Linda University Vegetarian Nutrition and Health Letter (www.llu.edu/llu/vegetarian).

Melina, Vesanto, Brenda Davis, and Victoria Harrison. *Becoming Vegetarian: The Complete Guide to Adopting a Vegetarian Diet.* Summertown, Tenn.: Book Publishing Co., 1995.

Moosewood Collective. *Moosewood Low-Fat Favorites.* New York: Clarkson Potter, 1996.

Nutrition Action Health Letter (Center for Science in the Public Interest, Washington, D.C., www.cspinet.org).

Spitler, Sue. *1001 Low-Fat Vegetarian Recipes,* 2nd ed. Chicago: Surrey Books, 2000.

Ornish, Dean. *Eat More, Weight Less.* New York: HarperPerennial, 1993.

Ornish, Dean. *Everyday Cooking with Dr. Dean Ornish.* New York: HarperCollins, 1997.

Tufts University Health and Nutrition Letter (www.healthletter.tufts.edu).

Vegetarian Times Low-Fat and Fast. New York: Macmillan, 1997.

Cyberdiet (www.cyberdiet.com).

Food and Nutrition Information Center (www.nal.usda.gov/fnic).

InteliHealth (www.intelihealth.com).

International Food Information Council Foundation (www.ificinfo.health.org).

Veg Source (www.vegsource.com).

RESOURCES FROM THE AMERICAN YOGA ASSOCIATION

Further information on Yoga is available from the American Yoga Association. To obtain free information about Yoga, including a complete catalog and guidelines for choosing a qualified teacher, visit our web site or send a self-addressed envelope stamped with postage for two ounces to the following address:

American Yoga Association
P.O. Box 19986
Sarasota, FL 34276

If you have a specific question about Yoga and would like a personal reply, write to the address above or contact us by telephone, fax, or e-mail:

Telephone: (941) 927-4977
Fax: (941) 921-9844
E-mail: info@americanyogaassociation.org
Web site: www.americanyogaassociation.org

We offer classes in the Cleveland, Ohio, area. For more information, write or call:

American Yoga Association
P.O. Box 18105
Cleveland Heights, OH 44106
Telephone: (216) 556-1313

Books

The American Yoga Association's Easy Does It Yoga (New York: Fireside/Simon & Schuster, 1999). For those with physical limitations, this book includes instruction in specially adapted Yoga exercises that can be done in a chair or in bed, breathing techniques, and meditation.

The American Yoga Association Wellness Book (New York: Kensington Books, 1996). A basic routine to maintain health and well-being, plus chapters on how Yoga can help specifically with arthritis, heart disease, back pain, PMS and menopause, weight management, insomnia, headaches, and eight other health conditions.

The American Yoga Association's New Yoga Challenge (Lincolnwood, Ill.: NTC Contemporary, 1997). Routines for energy, strength, flexibility, focus, and stability offer more vigorous Yoga workouts for body and mind. The last chapter, "The Powerful Individual," teaches you how to design your own routine.

The American Yoga Association's Yoga for Sports (Lincolnwood, Ill.: NTC Contemporary Books, 2000). A comprehensive book for every athlete, including techniques for bringing the physical and emotional-spiritual bodies together to attain peak performance. Includes a core routine of exercise, breathing, and meditation, plus specific exercise routines for dozens of individual sports, team sports, and coaches.

Arthritis: An American Yoga Association Wellness Guide (New York: Kensington Books, 2001). A complete program for management of osteo- and rheumatoid arthritis in six parts: Yoga exercise, breathing, and meditation, combined with fantasy techniques, a special walking program, diet and nutrition recommendations, and advice on alternative therapies.

Conversations with Swami Lakshmanjoo, Volume I: Aspects of Kashmir Shaivism (Sarasota, Fla.: American Yoga Association, 1995). Edited transcripts of Alice Christensen's interviews with Swami Lakshmanjoo, talking about his childhood and early years in Yoga, plus some basic concepts in the philosophy of Kashmir Shaivism.

Conversations with Swami Lakshmanjoo, Volume II: The Yamas and Niyamas of Patanjali (Sarasota, Fla.: American Yoga Association, 1998). Edited transcripts of Alice Christensen's dialogues with Swami Lakshmanjoo about these essential ethical guidelines in Yoga.

The Easy Does It Yoga Trainer's Guide (Dubuque, Iowa: Kendall-Hunt, 1995). A complete manual for how to begin teaching the Easy Does It Yoga program to adults with physical limitations due to age, convalescence, substance abuse, injury, or obesity. Excellent for health professionals, activities directors, physical therapists, home health aides, and others who work with the elderly or in rehabilitative services.

Heart Health: An American Yoga Association Wellness Guide (New York: Kensington Books, 2001). A complete program for either preventing or reversing heart disease, encompassing Yoga techniques of exercise, breathing, meditation, and fantasy, combined with aerobic walking and up-to-date nutrition advice.

The Light of Yoga (Sarasota, Fla.: American Yoga Association, 1970, 1978, 1997). A chronicle of the unusual circumstances that catapulted Alice Christensen into Yoga practice in the early 1950s, including the teachers and experiences that shaped her first years of study.

Meditation (Sarasota, Fla.: American Yoga Association, 1994). A collection of excerpts from lectures and classes on the subject of meditation, including a section of questions and answers from students.

20-Minute Yoga Workouts (New York: Ballantine, 1995). Brief routines that anyone can fit into the busiest schedule. Includes chapters on women's issues, toning and shaping, the "20-minute challenge," and workouts to do when you're away from home.

Reflections of Love (Sarasota, Fla.: American Yoga Association, 1994). A collection of excerpts from Alice Christensen's lectures and classes on the subject of love.

Weight Management: An American Yoga Association Wellness Guide (New York: Kensington Books, 2001). A complete program for weight management in six parts: Yoga exercise, breathing, and meditation, combined with fantasy techniques, a special walking program, and a healthy and enjoyable diet plan.

Yoga of the Heart: Ten Ethical Principles for Gaining Limitless Growth, Confidence, and Achievement (New York: Daybreak/Rodale Books, 1998). A clear, direct presentation of ten essential ethics—Nonviolence, Truthfulness, Nonstealing, Celibacy, Nonhoarding, Purity, Contentment, Tolerance, Study, and Remembrance—that help a person realize the power and support of joining the physical and emotional-spiritual bodies. Each chapter includes suggestions for how to start practicing, common pitfalls, and many examples from students' experiences and from mythology to illustrate the journey.

Audiotapes

Complete Relaxation and Meditation with Alice Christensen. A two-tape program that features three guided meditation sessions of varying lengths, including instruction in a seated posture, plus a discussion of meditation experiences.

The "I Love You" Meditation Technique. This technique begins with the experience of a more conscious connection with the breath through love. It then extends this feeling throughout the body and mind in relaxation and meditation. This tape teaches you the beauty of loving yourself and removes unseen fear.

Videotapes

Basic Yoga. A complete introduction to Yoga that includes exercise, breathing, and relaxation and meditation techniques. Provides detailed instruction in all the techniques, including variations for more or less flexibility, plus a special limbering routine and back-strengthening exercises. Features a 30-minute daily routine demonstrated in a Yoga class.

Conversations with Swami Lakshmanjoo. A set of three videotapes in which Alice Christensen introduces Swami Lakshmanjoo and talks with him about his background, the philosophy of Kashmir Shaivism, and other topics in Yoga. (Some material corresponds to the book *Conversations with Swami Lakshmanjoo, Volume I: Aspects of Kashmir Shaivism.*)

The Yamas and Niyamas: A Videotape Study Program. A set of twenty-five videotapes of Alice Christensen's comprehensive lectures on the ethical guidelines that form the cornerstone of Yoga philosophy and practice.

The Hero in Yoga: A Videotape Study Program. A series of twenty-four videotaped lectures by Alice Christensen on Joseph Campbell's landmark text *The Hero with a Thousand Faces,* showing how the adventure of the hero, represented in mythologies all over the globe, parallels the Yoga student's search for self-actualization.

Index

3⁵⁰ 03/13